CW00665917

We Can't Spell Success Without YOU

Brand Versus Brand
The Book
2019 Heart & Cholesterol Edition

We Can't Spell Success Without You

Brand Versus Brand the Book

2019 Heart & Cholesterol Edition

ISBN 978-1-9999425-4-0

WECANTSPELLSUCCESSWITHOUTYOU@GMAIL.COM

Or visit one of our websites for further information.

WWW.NADIET.INFO

WWW.WECANTSPELLSUCCESSWITHOUTYOU.COM

Preface

This book intends to help all people who struggle with heart and cholesterol issues, who have encountered diets in the past and they have not worked, and people who are subject to illnesses or poor health due to their current lifestyle.

A great solution to these problems is to read the We Can't Spell S ccess Without YOU – PowerPlan, this book is available as either a Gold or Silver edition. When using these books, some people could feel that a little extra help is required when purchasing their favourite food on a daily basis. This book simply provides a solution by being a more convenient method of providing this information when shopping.

This book simply lists all the food types in order so you are able to select the correct brand to achieve the **new you** while shopping. All the brands listed are available on our websites in downloadable fact sheets, but this can be inconvenient when actively shopping. In addition, selecting the correct brand for your health needs becomes difficult if the internet signal on your device is slow or even lost while selecting your favourite foods.

This book is optional when using the PowerPlan lifestyle change, but is a great and convenient reference where details of food brands are in one place. This simply allows you to make better branded food choices while shopping,

If the food brand you like is not listed in this book, then email and let us know. We are happy to create a new fact sheet and added to our website.

Disclaimer

Details of food listed in this book were correct at the time when the information was collected. Downloading fact sheets from www.nadiet.info will show the actual date the information is collected.

Some websites and supermarkets fail to show nutrition information for the foods that they sell. In this circumstance, further research is required to determine the product's nutritional value using google, galaxy health and my fitness pal to obtain the correct information.

Some food types will show nutrition information in millilitres (ml) and others in grams (g) for the identical type of food. Obtaining a more meaningful comparison is achieved by converting the ml liquid to grams based on the liquid weight. In these instances, the grams weight has been chosen as you are more likely to weigh food using grams when calorie counting.

If you are using the information on our website, there is no need to purchase this book unless you require the information that is conveniently printed rather than free online. This printed version provides a permanent record of food size, nutritional information and price during 2019, PRE-BREXIT, in the UK.

During the progress of time the website will be updated, without notification, with revised brands, food size, nutritional information and price. This information will be used to create revised versions of this book in future years.

Brand Placements

Please be aware this book uses unpaid branded products. I am not receiving any money to review these products. Any recommendation to purchase a type of food brand is due to its nutritional value and price rather than brand identity.

Contents

Introduction

This book is for people who want to control heart and cholesterol issues. Each section focuses on a type of food, for example vegetables, canned food, sauces, etc.

Every type of food has a subcategory so you can find the products quickly. For example, vegetables will include carrots, apples, onions, etc. as a subcategory.

All foods in this book are organised in saturated fat order, if you need to reduce your internal bad fat levels then select a brand of food from the top of each list.

If the best brand shown is not available at your local supermarket then simply choose the next one in the list until you are able to purchase your product.

If you find that the best brand for your circumstances is simply not appealing, the next time you are shopping then select the next on the list. Eventually you will find the brand that you will really like, that will help you control your heart and cholesterol issues, and will remove any deprived feelings that you will normally have when using a diabetic diet!

If you find that the brands that you need to purchase are simply not at your local supermarket then consider switching to a healthier shop. This, over time, due to loss in profits will encourage supermarkets to sell food that is healthier for us rather than making massive profits for the store. No supermarket wants to lose custom as they could possibly go out of business.

When finding the food brand in a supermarket that is not labelled with calorie and nutrition information then don't purchase or eat it. Simply find another brand or decided on an alternative favourite food that you like, even better learn how to cook the meal yourself at home that will be far healthier, will increase your culinary skills and provide you with a new hobby that everyone in your family will enjoy.

Over time these books will show if calories, saturated fats and carbohydrates are being reduced that will result in us eating more natural and healthier food from the supermarket. If calorie, saturated fat and carbohydrates are increased then the foods are becoming less healthy and more tampered with the intention to increase supermarkets and shops profits.

Finally, these books will show if the food weight and price are static over time. If the weight of the food is reduced and the price is the same or higher than we are paying more for the food and have a less financial budget for our families. Likewise, if the weight of the food increases or remains the same where the price is unchanged or reduced, then we are paying less for our food. This allows everyone to meet their family's needs easier within their financial budget.

Other Publications
This book is designed to look at heart and cholesterol control, other similar books will be available in 2020 that supports the following:

Diabetes Type 2 Edition
Designed for people who are worried about, or who suffer with, Diabetes Type 2 in their life. This book is presented in the same manner as this edition, where all food brands are organised in carbohydrate order.

Weight Control Edition
Designed for people who are worried about, or who suffer with, weight issues in their life. This book is presented in the same manner as this edition, where all food brands are organised in calorie order.

Super Money Saver Edition
Designed for people who are worried about money daily who need to control a tight budget. This book is presented in the same manner as

this edition, where all food brands are organised by price order. This allows the reader to select the cheapest brands while shopping!

Time to Finally Control Your Bad Fats

Let us look in detail at this quick reference book. If you use the index at the front of the book to find the food you need to purchase, you will discover your best brands. This book is not a page-to-page read, although this will allow you to discover surprising food facts and prices!

Structure of This Book

This book will show you the food types and give my personal views and advice. Each food type has a subcategory making it is easy to find the food you like using the contents at the front of this book. All brands of food are organised as tables that are written in the following manner:

Suggested Brands

The name of the food brand is in the first Colum and shown as it appears on the product packaging. The product name appears exactly as the supermarkets have stored the food name. This includes the brand name and any miss-spelt wording shown on their shopping websites. This makes it easier to find the brand when shopping in the supermarket or on-line where you can identify the correct brand for your needs.

Size

The second column shows the size of the brand as an abbreviation as g for grams for solid food and ml for millilitre for liquid. When the product is a collection of the same item, this column shows the number of items. The higher this number means you will receive more food or drink for the price shown.

Kcal (Calories)

The third Colum shows the number of calories in the brand, abbreviated as Kcal. The lower this number the fewer calories, or energy, are in the food that will result in weight loss. The higher this number the more calories, or energy, are in the food that will lead to weight gain.

S. Fat (Saturated Fat)

The fourth Colum shows the amount of saturated fat in the brand, abbreviated as g for grams. The lower this number the better the food if you are concerned about blood pressure, heart, stroke and cholesterol issues. If you want to increase your weight, you can select the higher calorie product with the lower saturated fat. This allows you to gain weight without the worry of increased illnesses.

Carbs (Carbohydrates)

The fifth Colum shows the amount of carbohydrates in the brand, abbreviated as g for grams. The lower this number the better the food if you are concerned about diabetes type 2 issues. If you want to gain weight, you can select the higher calorie product with lower carbohydrates so you are able to gain weight without the worry of aggravating the diabetes type 2 condition or suffering from additional health issues.

£ (Price)

The final column shows the price of the food when logged in this book, you can find out the exact date by downloading and looking at the bottom of the fact sheet in the brand verses brand section of our website. This is also a good indication if the food price and size has changed and how it influences our pockets and eating habits over time.

Serving Size

At the bottom of each table, for every food type, there is a suggested serving size. The number of calories, saturated fat and carbohydrate shown in the table reflects this quantity of food. It is an excellent idea to weigh your food when using this book as 100 grams of a product can seem surprisingly small.

Product Exclusions

When writing this book some branded foods was excluded due to the calorie and nutrition information being unavailable. Some supermarkets fail to load their own branded products on their supermarket website, it becomes almost impossible to find the calorie and nutrition information without visiting the local store.

There is no explanation why supermarkets act in this manner, however, it seems to be a trend in 2019 with Morrison's leading the way with their M Saver range. The question is WHY, surely this supermarket will be losing thousands, if not millions, of pounds in lost sales!

Health and Wealth?

You can use this book to determine if you can improve your wealth along with your Health. This is achievable by visiting our website, WWW.NADIET.INFO, and clicking on downloads.

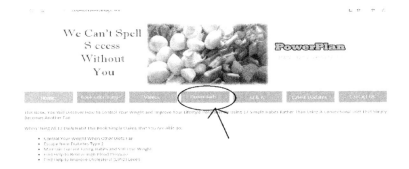

Click on the **Health and Wealth Savings Calculator** that will open a spreadsheet:

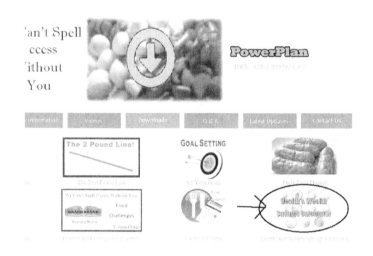

Assuming we are interested in Pizza on page 100, look down the list for your favourite brand. For example, The Pizza Express Margherita 12" that cost a bargain £3.00! This pizza you love so much you will eat it around twice a week, especially if there is a special event or you are having a late night at the weekend.

Suggested Brands	Size (g)	Kcal	S.fat (g)	Carbs (g)	£
Pizza Express Margherita 12"	455	1019.2	17.7	121.0	3.00

The table above, on page 110, shows our pizza brand with its nutrition information and price. We can enter this information into the **Health and Wealth Savings Calculator** spreadsheet that was downloaded earlier.

Food Name: Pizza

Normal Brand: Pizza Express Margherita 12"

	Size (g)	Calories (Kcal)	Saturated Fat (g)	Carboydrate (g)	Price (£0.00)
	455	1019.2	17.7	121.0	£3.00

Revised Brand:

	Size (g)	Calories (Kcal)	Saturated Fat (g)	Carboydrate (g)	Price (£0.00)

Times Eaten Per Week:

Revisiting the list of pizzas on page 100, we can start from the top selecting a healthier alternative. Many healthier product options can be reduced in size, this will not matter if you are using the stomach tonic as described in the **We Can't Spell S ccess Without You - PowerPlan** (silver or gold edition) book.

Looking at the list, and because ASDA is an easy to find and popular supermarket, we have decided to purchase the ASDA Cheese & Tomato Pizza. This costs less than the Pizza Express Margherita and contains far less calories per pizza when compared to the favourite brand.

Suggested Brands	Size (g)	Kcal	S.fat (g)	Carbs (g)	£
ASDA Cheese & Tomato Pizza	110	294.8	3.6	40.7	0.61

We can add this nutritional and price information to the **Health and Wealth Savings Calculator** spreadsheet, along with the number of times per week that the pizza is eaten …. Twice ☺

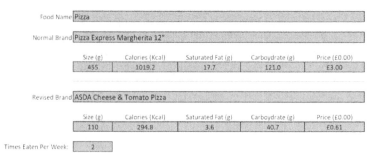

Food Name: Pizza

Normal Brand: Pizza Express Margherita 12"

Size (g)	Calories (Kcal)	Saturated Fat (g)	Carboydrate (g)	Price (£0.00)
455	1019.2	17.7	121.0	£3.00

Revised Brand: ASDA Cheese & Tomato Pizza

Size (g)	Calories (Kcal)	Saturated Fat (g)	Carboydrate (g)	Price (£0.00)
110	294.8	3.6	40.7	£0.61

Times Eaten Per Week: 2

Once this information has been added, the lower half of the spreadsheet will automatically show the benefits of the brand switch and your new choice.

Your Results	
Will My Food Amount Change?	**You Will Eat Less Food**
Will My Weight Change?	**You Will Lose Weight**
Is This Switch Good For Diabetes?	**Will Improve Over Time**
Is This Switch Good For The Heart?	**Will Improve Over Time**
Sugar Equivilant Change Yearly:	**-1670.24 Tea Spoons Less**
Price Change Over a Year:	**£248.56 Saved**
Perdicted Weight Change:	**-125.56 Pounds Lost**

This is a good indication of how your health will improve by switching brands rather than feeling deprived using a diet and avoiding the food completely. We can see that we would eat less pizza and would expect to lose weight over a year.

The new pizza option will also improve heart and cholesterol issues over time, as we would be eating only 3.6 grams of saturated fat compared to the original brand that contained 17.7 grams that is a lot considering maximum allowance is 30 grams for man or 20 grams for a women without any health issues. The trick is to select brand where you are able to eat little saturated fat as possible to improve your condition.

This reduced sugar and fats would result in a weight loss of 125.5 pounds in body weight per year by simply switching the pizza brand. This is a great achievement for people who suffer from health issues, and this single brand switch will also allow you to save £248.56 per year on the shopping bill.

You could conclude that this brand switch is not good for you as the size of the pizza is too small, you do not shop for groceries at Asda or you simply do not like the taste.

Based on these feelings you could try the **Pizza Express Vegan Giardiniera** that is also on the list on page 100.

Suggested Brands	Size (g)	Kcal	S.fat (g)	Carbs (g)	£
Pizza Express Vegan Giardiniera	272	549.4	7.9	82.4	5.00

This is a bigger pizza and the trade name, Pizza Express, will be more appealing to you as this is your favourite brand.

Enter the details of this pizza in the **Health and Wealth Savings Calculator** spreadsheet replacing the previously selected ASDA Cheese & Tomato Pizza.

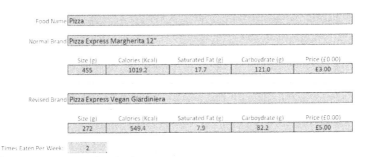

Food Name: Pizza

Normal Brand: Pizza Express Margherita 12"

Size (g)	Calories (Kcal)	Saturated Fat (g)	Carboydrate (g)	Price (£0.00)
455	1019.2	17.7	121.0	£3.00

Revised Brand: Pizza Express Vegan Giardiniera

Size (g)	Calories (Kcal)	Saturated Fat (g)	Carboydrate (g)	Price (£0.00)
272	549.4	7.9	82.2	£5.00

Times Eaten Per Week: 2

Once you have updated the spreadsheet, the lower half will automatically refresh providing the following information for the revised brand choice.

Your Results		
Will My Food Amount Change?	You Will Eat Less Food	
Will My Weight Change?	You Will Lose Weight	
Is This Switch Good For Diabetes?	Will Improve Over Time	
Is This Switch Good For The Heart?	Will Improve Over Time	
Sugar Equivilant Change Yearly:	-807.04	Tea Spoons Less
Price Change Over a Year:	£208.00	Extra To Spend
Perdicted Weight Change:	-81.43	Pounds Lost

The result are very similar, switching to this pizza also will improve your overall health. You will improve your heart and cholesterol as you be eating only 7.9 grams of saturated fat compared to the original brand that contained 17.7 grams, also we would be eating around 807 teaspoons less sugar from the food that is stored as either pure sugar or carbohydrate resulting in your HAb1c lowering.

Keeping your favourite brand but switching to a healthier product will result in you paying £208 more per year. This can be a small price to pay when improving health and fitness BUT there are many other products to try that are cheaper and better for you, the trick is finding the brand that suits your budget and your health needs that you really like to eat!

Vegetables

Always remember when choosing your vegetables

- If you purchase them from the supermarket you need to eat 7 per day

- If you purchase them from markets or local farms you need to eat 6 per day

- If you purchase them from Organic outlets you need to eat 5 per day

These figures are based on the nutritional value of the food and the daily body requirements.

Tomatoes are a great food that help to increase your resistance to cancer along with Broccoli, Sprouts, Carrots and Celery.

If you are taking a statin type medication, please avoid grapefruits completely. Digesting a small amount of grapefruit can stop the statin medication from working leading to high cholesterol, high blood pressure and possible stroke or heart attack. This is also true of grapefruit juice, where as little as 20 ml can stop the drug from working!

Apples

Suggested Brands	Size (pack)	Kcal	S.fat (g)	Carbs (g)	£
Supermarket Fresh	4	47	0.1	12	2.00
Locally Grown / Market	4	49	0.1	11.8	1.50
Organic Fresh	6	53	0.1	11.6	1.98

VALUES SHOWN PER 100 GRAMS SERVING

Banana

Suggested Brands	Size (pack)	Kcal	S.fat (g)	Carbs (g)	£
Locally Grown / Market	5	78	0.02	18	1.00
Organic Fresh	5	84	0.02	20.3	1.15
Supermarket Fresh	10	84	0.02	20	1.59
Budget Frozen	5	62	0.1	15.3	0.90

VALUES SHOWN PER 100 GRAMS SERVING

Broccoli

Suggested Brands	Size (g)	Kcal	S.fat (g)	Carbs (g)	£
Locally Grown / Market	300	34	0.02	2.8	0.80
Budget Frozen	1000	34	0.02	2.8	0.90
Supermarket Frozen	1000	34	0.02	2.8	0.95
Supermarket Fresh	360	34	0.1	2.8	0.58
Organic Fresh	300	34	0.1	2.8	1.00

VALUES SHOWN PER 100 GRAMS SERVING

Cabbage (White)

Suggested Brands	Size (g)	Kcal	S.fat (g)	Carbs (g)	£
Supermarket Frozen	750	21	0.0	2.3	0.95
Organic Fresh	1000	22	0.0	2.8	2.00
Locally Grown / Market	1000	24	0.0	3.4	1.30
Supermarket Fresh	1200	30	0.1	4.8	0.78

VALUES SHOWN PER 100 GRAMS SERVING

Carrots

Suggested Brands	Size (g)	Kcal	S.fat (g)	Carbs (g)	£
Budget Frozen	1000	28	0.1	4.4	1.00
Supermarket Frozen	900	28	0.1	4.4	1.00
Supermarket Fresh	500	35	0.2	6.0	0.35
Organic Fresh	500	35	0.2	6.0	0.58
Locally Grown / Market	500	35	0.2	5.5	0.60

VALUES SHOWN PER 100 GRAMS SERVING

Celery

Suggested Brands	Size (g)	Kcal	S.fat (g)	Carbs (g)	£
Supermarket Fresh	450	10	0.02	0.9	0.60
Locally Grown / Market	400	10	0.02	0.9	0.70
Organic Fresh	350	10	0.02	0.9	1.00

VALUES SHOWN PER 100 GRAMS SERVING

Grapefruit

Suggested Brands	Size (g)	Kcal	S.fat (g)	Carbs (g)	£
Sainsbury's White Grapefruit	100	34	0.0	6.8	0.55
Sainsbury's Red Grapefruit	100	34	0.0	6.8	0.60
Pink Grapefruit (each)	100	34	0.0	6.8	0.70
Organic	100	40	0.0	10.00	1.25

VALUES SHOWN PER 100 GRAMS SERVING

Green (Pigeon) Peas

Suggested Brands	Size (g)	Kcal	S.fat (g)	Carbs (g)	£
Organic Fresh	500	81	0.09	10.7	1.59
Supermarket Frozen	1000	83	0.09	11	0.99
Budget Frozen	1000	84	0.09	11	0.72
Locally Grown / Market	500	88	0.09	10	1.00
Birds Eye	800	68	0.1	7.5	2.00
Supermarket Fresh	160	90	0.3	10	0.95

VALUES SHOWN PER 100 GRAMS SERVING

Leeks

Suggested Brands	Size (g)	Kcal	S.fat (g)	Carbs (g)	£
Budget Frozen	175	24	0.02	2.5	0.60
Locally Grown / Market	500	25	0.02	2.7	1.00
Supermarket Frozen	700	26	0.02	2.6	0.95
Organic Fresh	400	27	0.02	2.8	2.25
Supermarket Fresh	500	25	0.1	2.6	1.00

VALUES SHOWN PER 100 GRAMS SERVING

Mushrooms (White)

Suggested Brands	Size (g)	Kcal	S.fat (g)	Carbs (g)	£
Organic Fresh	300	8	0.1	0.4	1.00
Locally Grown / Market	300	12	0.1	0.4	0.80
Supermarket Fresh	300	16	0.1	0.4	0.95
Supermarket Frozen	500	41	0.2	5.8	2.00
Budget Frozen	600	108	0.8	0.4	0.95

VALUES SHOWN PER 100 GRAMS SERVING

Onions (White / Brown)

Suggested Brands	Size (g)	Kcal	S.fat (g)	Carbs (g)	£
Supermarket Fresh	500	41	0.02	7.9	0.50
Locally Grown / Market	500	44	0.02	5.9	0.70
Organic Fresh	500	42	0.2	5.6	1.20
Supermarket Frozen	650	48	0.2	5.3	1.00
Budget Frozen	650	100	0.6	11	0.95

VALUES SHOWN PER 100 GRAMS SERVING

Potatoes

Suggested Brands	Size (g)	Kcal	S.fat (g)	Carbs (g)	£
Organic Fresh	1500	68	0.04	14.9	1.18
British Jazzy	1000	70	0.04	15.4	2.00
Buttery Marabel	2000	74	0.04	18	2.00
Albert Bartlett Rooster	2000	75	0.04	16	2.00
Selected Red	2500	77	0.04	18	1.60
White	2500	77	0.05	17.5	1.30
Maris Piper	2500	102	0.05	22.6	1.80
Sweet Potatoes	1000	95	0.1	20.5	1.00
Marabel Baking Potatoes	4 pack	97	0.1	23	1.20
King Edward	2500	166	0.7	26.4	1.80
Budget Frozen (mash)	900	98	1.2	17	0.90
Supermarket Frozen (mash)	650	96	1.6	16	1.45

VALUES SHOWN PER 100 GRAMS SERVING

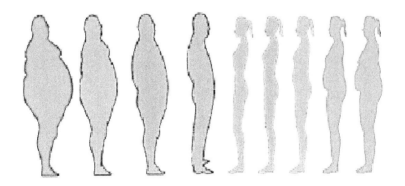

Sprouts

Suggested Brands	Size (g)	Kcal	S.fat (g)	Carbs (g)	£
Organic Fresh	300	24.0	0.1	1.9	1.30
Waitrose trimmed brussels sprouts	330	30.6	0.1	2.5	1.50
essential Waitrose Brussel sprouts	500	22.2	0.2	2.1	0.60
ASDA Grower's Selection Brussels Sprouts	300	24.6	0.2	2.1	1.25
Locally Grown / Market	200	25.2	0.2	2.1	1.00
Tesco Button Brussels Sprouts	1000	25.2	0.2	2.0	1.10
ASDA Trimmed Brussels Sprouts	200	25.8	0.2	2.1	1.00
ASDA Frozen for Freshness Brussels Sprouts	1000	26.4	0.2	2.1	0.99
Morrisons Button Sprouts	1000	26.4	0.2	1.5	1.00
Sainsbury's Button Sprouts	1000	26.4	0.2	2.1	1.30
Sainsbury's Brussels Sprouts	200	27.0	0.2	2.1	1.50
Morrisons Prepared Sprouts	250	30.0	0.2	2.3	1.60
Tesco Peeled Baby Sprouts	180	30.6	0.2	2.5	1.00
Redmere Farms Brussels Sprouts	300	30.6	0.2	2.5	1.00
Waitrose Baby Sprouts	300	30.6	0.2	2.5	1.00
Iceland Button Sprouts	900	30.6	0.2	2.5	1.00
Waitrose Trimmed baby sprouts	100	30.6	0.2	2.5	1.10

Vegetables Strawberry

Suggested Brands	Size (g)	Kcal	S.fat (g)	Carbs (g)	£
Tesco Peeled Brussels Sprouts	200	30.6	0.2	2.5	1.25
Good4U Super Sprouts	60	21.0	0.5	0.8	1.00

Values shown per 60 Grams Serving

Strawberry

Suggested Brands	Size (g)	Kcal	S.fat (g)	Carbs (g)	£
Supermarket Fresh	400	30	0.01	6	2.89
Locally Grown / Market	350	32	0.01	7	1.50
Organic Fresh	350	34	0.01	7.6	3.50

Values shown per 100 Grams Serving

Tomatoes

Suggested Brands	Size (g)	Kcal	S.fat (g)	Carbs (g)	£
Budget Canned	400	18	0.0	3.0	0.28
Supermarket Canned	400	25	0.05	3.8	0.35
Organic Fresh	4 Pack	16	0.1	3.0	1.60
Locally Grown / Market	600	18	0.1	3.1	1.20
Supermarket Fresh	750	20	0.1	3.1	1.15

Values shown per 100 Grams Serving

Common Food

Herbs and spices are generally calorie free making them handy when cooking meals at home. This allows you to create your own low calorie and enjoyable dish that is unique to yourself and will benefit your families' health.

When home cooking you know exactly what is in all the food that you eat. This allows you to control calories, saturated fat and carbohydrates to produce a healthier dish for you and your family.

Remember that bread slows down the digestive system; this allows all the food ate after the bread to leave the body at a much slower pace. This process results in the body storing excess calories, sugars and fats from the food along with the calorific bread that we have just eaten.

If you are worried about feeling hungry then substitute the bread with your favourite vegetable. This will ensure that you are not hungry during the day and is a much healthier alternative to bread.

Breakfast Items

Suggested Brands	Size	Kcal	S.fat (g)	Carbs (g)	£
Grilled Tomato	1 Item	10	0	1.6	n/a
Baked beans	½ Can	162	0.0	25.9	n/a
Canned tomatoes	½ Can	50	0.2	7.5	n/a
Toast	1 slice	96	0.2	18	n/a
Fried Tomato	1 Item	34	0.7	1.9	n/a
Fried Bread	1 slice	141	1.2	13.6	n/a
Poached Egg	1 egg	66	1.3	0.08	n/a
Back Bacon	2 slices	89	1.3	1.0	n/a
Mushrooms (Fried)	1 cup	77	1.5	8.3	n/a
Fried Egg	1 egg	90	2.0	0.4	n/a
Black Pudding	1 slice	108	2.1	6.7	n/a
White Pudding	1 slice	115	2.8	7.7	n/a
Scrambled Egg	1 egg	91	4.0	2.0	n/a
Pork Sausage	1 link	125	4.0	7.8	n/a

VALUES SHOWN PER SIZE DISPLAYED IN THE TABLE

Bread

Suggested Brands	Size (g)	Kcal	S.fat (g)	Carbs (g)	£
Sainsbury's Farmhouse White Bread	400	121	0.05	24.1	0.80
Sainsbury's Farmhouse Loaf White Bread	800	121	0.05	22.5	1.10
Sainsbury's Sandwich Loaf White Bread	800	121	0.05	24.1	1.10
Kingsmill No Crusts 50/50 Bread	400	47	0.1	8.5	1.40
Kingsmill No Crusts Soft White Bread	400	50	0.1	9.7	1.40
Weight Watchers Danish Malted Bread	400	51	0.1	9	0.99
Warburtons Wholemeal Medium Sliced Bread	400	55	0.1	9	0.90
Warburtons White Medium Sliced Bread	400	58	0.1	10.8	0.90
Warburtons White Danish Bread	400	63	0.1	11.8	0.90
Hovis Tasty Wholemeal Bread	400	64	0.1	11	0.85
ASDA Soft White Medium Sliced	400	68	0.1	13	0.45
Sainsbury's Wholemeal Bread Medium	400	68	0.1	10.8	0.50
Kingsmill 50/50 Medium Sliced Bread	400	68	0.1	12.2	0.80
Warburtons Toastie White Thick Sliced Bread	400	70	0.1	13.1	0.90

Suggested Brands	Size (g)	Kcal	S.fat (g)	Carbs (g)	£
Morrisons Medium Wholemeal Loaf	400	72	0.1	12.7	0.45
Sainsbury's Toastie Sliced White Bread	400	79	0.1	15.2	0.50
Morrisons Wholemeal Medium Loaf	800	79	0.1	13.8	0.55
Tesco Finest Super Grained Farmhouse Loaf	400	80	0.1	14.3	0.79
Daily's Medium Sliced Wholemeal Bread	800	83	0.1	14	0.45
Morrisons Medium White Loaf	800	84	0.1	16.2	0.55
Sainsbury's Medium Sliced Wholemeal Bread, SO Organic	400	85	0.1	14.4	0.90
Genius Gluten Free White Toastie Bread	500	85	0.1	15	2.70
Daily's Medium Sliced White Bread	800	86	0.1	16.3	0.45
Morrisons Wholemeal Toastie Loaf	800	91	0.1	16	0.55
Tesco Free From Sliced White Bread	550	92	0.1	15.8	1.80
Tesco Free From White Sliced Bread	400	92	0.1	17.2	1.80
Hovis Medium Soft White Bread	800	93	0.1	17.9	1.00
Crusty White Farmhouse Loaf Sliced	400	97	0.1	19	0.79
Crusty White Farmhouse Loaf	400	97	0.1	19	0.79

COMMON FOOD   BREAD

Suggested Brands	Size (g)	Kcal	S.fat (g)	Carbs (g)	£
Roberts Bakery Medium White Bread	800	97	0.1	18.9	1.05
Morrisons White Toastie Loaf	800	98	0.1	18.9	0.55
Iceland Thick Sliced Wholemeal Bread	800	101	0.1	17.8	0.79
Iceland Medium Tiger Bloomer Bread	800	101	0.1	19.6	1.00
Rathbones Farmhouse Loaf	400	102	0.1	19.8	0.62
Morrisons Toastie White With More	800	103	0.1	20	0.55
Tesco Finest White Loaf	800	104	0.1	20	0.99
Roberts Bakery Thick White Bread	800	113	0.1	22.1	1.05
Morrisons Super Toastie White Loaf	800	124	0.1	24	0.55
Kingsmill No Crusts Wholemeal Bread	400	45	0.2	7.4	1.40
Warburtons White Milk Roll Bread	400	46	0.2	8.3	0.90
Weight Watchers Thick Wholemeal Bread	400	64	0.2	11	1.14
ASDA Wholemeal Medium Sliced	400	67	0.2	10	0.46
essential Waitrose wholemeal medium sliced bread	800	74	0.2	12.3	0.60
Sainsbury's Multiseed Thick Sliced Wholemeal Bread, SO Organic	400	79	0.2	9.3	1.10

Suggested Brands	Size (g)	Kcal	S.fat (g)	Carbs (g)	£
Waitrose Ancient Grains & Oat Cob	600	83	0.2	14.9	1.29
Hovis Original Granary Bread	400	84	0.2	15.3	0.90
Waitrose Wholemeal Farmhouse Medium	800	84	0.2	14.2	1.30
Tesco Wholemeal Bread	440	85	0.2	13.9	0.50
Hovis Best of Both Medium Bread	750	86	0.2	15.2	1.00
Hovis Medium Wholemeal Bread	800	88	0.2	15.1	1.00
Hovis Seed Sensations Seven Seeds Bread	400	92	0.2	13.9	0.90
Sainsbury's Medium Sliced Wholemeal Bread	800	93	0.2	14.7	0.55
ASDA Square Cut Medium Wholemeal Bread	800	93	0.2	15	0.55
Tesco Wholemeal Medium Bread	800	93	0.2	14.7	0.59
Rathbones Medium White Loaf	800	93	0.2	16.9	0.80
Kingsmill Tasty Medium Wholemeal Bread	800	93	0.2	15.4	1.10
Kingsmill Medium 50/50 Bread	800	94	0.2	16.8	1.10
ASDA Square Cut Medium White Bread	800	96	0.2	18	0.55
Sainsbury's Soft Medium Sliced White Bread	800	96	0.2	18.2	0.55
Tesco White Medium Bread	800	96	0.2	18.2	0.59

COMMON FOOD   BREAD

Suggested Brands	Size (g)	Kcal	S.fat (g)	Carbs (g)	£
Tesco Finest Wholemeal Loaf	800	97	0.2	16.2	0.99
Waitrose soft white medium sliced	800	97	0.2	18.1	1.00
Warburtons Medium White Bread	800	98	0.2	18.7	1.10
Warburtons Old English White	400	99	0.2	17.7	1.25
Tesco Wholemeal Farmhouse Loaf	800	103	0.2	16.8	0.79
Tesco Wholemeal Farmhouse Loaf	800	103	0.2	16.8	0.79
ASDA Extra Special Farmhouse Wholemeal & Rye Bread	800	103	0.2	17	0.84
Warburtons Medium Wholemeal Bread	800	103	0.2	16.9	1.10
Kingsmill Thick 50/50 Bread	800	103	0.2	18.4	1.10
Hovis Thick Wholemeal Bread	800	104	0.2	17.8	1.00
Warburtons Farmhouse Soft White Bread	800	104	0.2	19.2	1.00
Brace's Family Bread Luxury Medium White Sliced Bread	800	104	0.2	21.2	1.00
Hovis Granary Wholemeal Bread	800	104	0.2	17.5	1.40
Tesco White Farmhouse Loaf	800	106	0.2	20.1	0.79

Common Food   Bread

Suggested Brands	Size (g)	Kcal	S.fat (g)	Carbs (g)	£
Rathbone Wholemeal Toastie	800	106	0.2	19.2	0.80
Morrisons The Best Thick Cut Malted Grain Loaf	800	106	0.2	18.7	1.00
Tesco Finest Super Grained Farmhouse Sproutedrye	800	106	0.2	19.1	1.10
Allinson's The Champion Wholemeal Bread	650	108	0.2	17.4	1.65
Rathbones Toastie Bread White	800	109	0.2	19.7	0.80
ASDA Extra Special Farmhouse White Bread	800	109	0.2	21	0.89
Tesco Finest Oat & Barley Loaf	800	109	0.2	19.8	1.10
Hovis Seed Sensations Wholemeal Bread	800	109	0.2	13.8	1.50
Morrisons The Best Ancient Grain Loaf	400	111	0.2	19.3	0.75
Mothers Pride Scottish Plain Medium	800	115	0.2	21.9	1.00
Warburtons Toastie White Bread	800	116	0.2	22	1.10
Waitrose Soft White Farmhouse	800	116	0.2	22.2	1.30
Waitrose Duchy Organic wholemeal batch	800	116	0.2	20.3	1.65
Hovis Thick Soft White Bread	800	117	0.2	22.3	1.00

Suggested Brands	Size (g)	Kcal	S.fat (g)	Carbs (g)	£
Brace's Family Bread Luxury Thick White Sliced Bread	800	117	0.2	23.7	1.00
Tesco Multigrain Batch	800	120	0.2	21.8	0.79
Warburtons Lancashire Thorough Bread	800	120	0.2	22	1.00
Waitrose farmhouse batch multigrain	800	120	0.2	22.5	1.45
Waitrose Soft White Thick Bread	800	121	0.2	22.6	1.00
Malted Grain Loaf Sliced	800	125	0.2	23.5	1.10
Tiger Loaf Sliced	800	126	0.2	24.3	1.10
Crusty White Sandwich Loaf Sliced	800	128	0.2	25.3	1.10
Crusty White Sandwich Loaf	800	128	0.2	25.3	1.10
Tesco Crusty White Farmhouse Loaf Sliced	800	128	0.2	25.3	1.10
Hovis Extra Thick Soft White Bread	800	156	0.2	29.9	1.00
Roberts Bakery Mega Thick White Bread	800	156	0.2	30.4	1.05
Tesco Finest High Protein Loaf	400	84	0.3	10.5	0.85
Tesco Multiseed Loaf	400	88	0.3	13.3	0.59
Waitrose Sunflower & Pumpkin Cob	600	89	0.3	13	1.29
Vogel Seeded Wholemeal Bread	800	100	0.3	12	1.55
Vogel's Soya & Linseed Medium Sliced Bread	800	101	0.3	14	1.55

Suggested Brands	Size (g)	Kcal	S.fat (g)	Carbs (g)	£
Wonderloaf Medium	800	103	0.3	18.3	1.00
Kingsmill Tasty Thick Wholemeal Bread	800	103	0.3	17	1.10
Waitrose Wholemeal Farmhouse Thick	800	103	0.3	17.4	1.30
Sainsbury's Thick Sliced Wholemeal Bread	800	104	0.3	16.3	0.55
Kingsmill Thick Soft White Bread	800	105	0.3	20.1	1.10
Tesco Free From Sliced Seeded Bread	550	107	0.3	14.5	2.10
Hovis Thick Granary Bread	800	112	0.3	20.4	1.45
Morrisons The Best Seeded Loaf	800	114	0.3	16.7	1.00
Sainsbury's Thick Sliced Wholemeal Bread, SO Organic	800	119	0.3	19.7	1.45
Sainsbury's Toastie Thick Sliced White Bread	800	120	0.3	22.8	0.55
ASDA Soft White Toastie Thick Sliced	800	120	0.3	23	0.55
Tesco Toastie White Thick Slice	800	120	0.3	22.8	0.59
Hovis Seed Sensations Seven Seeds Bread	800	131	0.3	19.7	1.50
Warburtons Thickest White Bread	800	140	0.3	26.7	1.10
Iceland White Bloomer Bread	800	158	0.3	28.1	1.00

COMMON FOOD   BREAD

Suggested Brands	Size (g)	Kcal	S.fat (g)	Carbs (g)	£
Brace's Family Bread Luxury Doorstep White Sliced Bread	800	166	0.3	28.7	1.00
essential Waitrose white medium sliced bread	800	83	0.4	15.3	0.60
Warburtons Seeded Batch Bread	400	85	0.4	11.6	0.95
Hi-Lo Seeded Medium Sliced Wholemeal Bread	400	86	0.4	5	1.75
Morrisons The Best Oat & Barley Loaf	800	110	0.4	18.8	1.00
Morrisons The Best Wholemeal Sunflower Seed & Spelt Farmhouse	800	113	0.4	16.6	1.00
Tesco Finest Dark Rye& Sunflower	600	115	0.4	17.2	0.99
Wonderloaf Thick	800	122	0.4	21.7	1.00
Morrisons The Best Sunflower & Pumpkin Seed Loaf	800	123	0.4	16.9	1.00
Tesco Multiseed Batch	800	133	0.4	20.2	0.79
Morrisons The Best Soya & Linseed Loaf	800	116	0.5	16.7	1.00
Morrisons The Best Seeded Loaf	400	119	0.5	17.5	0.75
Tesco Finest Super Seeded Farmhouse	800	130	0.5	16.7	1.10
ASDA Extra Special Super Seeded Bread	800	131	0.5	17	0.84

Suggested Brands	Size (g)	Kcal	S.fat (g)	Carbs (g)	£
Brace's Family Bread 50% White & Wholemeal Thick Sliced Bread	800	131	0.5	24.6	1.00
Iceland Seeded Bloomer Bread	800	152	0.5	20.8	1.00
Iceland Thick Tiger Bloomer Bread	800	168	0.5	27.5	1.00
Hovis Nimble Wholemeal Bread	400	51	0.6	8.1	0.85
Hovis Lower Carb Deliciously Seeded Bread	400	98	0.6	9.9	1.20
Morrisons The Best Sunflower & Pumpkin Seed Loaf	400	122	0.6	17.1	0.75
Tesco Finest Sunflower & Pumpkin Loaf	600	127	0.6	16.2	0.99
Warburtons Seeded Batch Bread	800	134	0.6	18.2	1.60
Sainsbury's Soft Multiseed Farmhouse Thick Sliced Wholemeal Bread, Taste the Difference	800	140	0.6	16.9	1.10
Waitrose Farmhouse Batch Multiseed	800	146	0.6	19.2	1.45
Burgen Soya & Linseed Bread	800	126	0.7	11.8	1.30
Sainsbury's Sunflower Seeded Medium Sliced Rye Bread Bloomer, Taste the Difference	400	181	0.7	20.5	1.50

Common Food   Cakes

Suggested Brands	Size (g)	Kcal	S.fat (g)	Carbs (g)	£
Sainsbury's Sunflower & Pumpkin, Taste the Difference	800	155	0.8	18.3	1.10

Values shown per Slice of Bread

Cakes

Suggested Brands	Size (Pack)	Kcal	S.fat (g)	Carbs (g)	£
Plain Fairy Cakes	X 12	88	0.4	10.8	1.15
Iced Fairy Cakes	X 12	100	0.6	13.7	1.15
Chocolate Brownie with Himalayan Rose Salt	X 1	165	1.9	17	2.05
Flapjack	X 5	146	2.1	20	1.00
Choco Honey Snack Cakes	X 10	98	2.3	14.2	1.00
Classic Milk Snack Cakes	X 10	99	2.4	14.3	1.00
Almond Fingers	X 4	183	2.7	27.9	1.00
Bramley Apple Pies	X6	212	2.7	32.8	1.00
Congress Tart	X 4	196	3	30.3	1.34
Cherry Bakewell Tart	X 4	308	3.2	52.7	1.34
Mince Pies	X 6	204	3.3	32.3	1.00
Custard Donuts	X 2	213	3.3	10	1.25
Indulgent Cupcakes	X12	213	3.5	26	4.00
Fresh Cream Sponge Cake	6 "	138	4.1	18.2	2.00
Fresh Cream Chocolate Sponge	6 "	137	4.5	15.4	2.00
Egg Custard Tart	X 2	242	4.5	29.9	0.80
Chorley Cakes	X 4	286	4.5	37.5	1.20
Fresh Cream Lemon Sponge	6 "	143	4.6	18.3	2.00
Vanilla Custard Slice	X 2	290	5.2	41.2	1.65

COMMON FOOD CAKES

Suggested Brands	Size (Pack)	Kcal	S.fat (g)	Carbs (g)	£
Chocolate Éclairs	X 2	216	7	16.7	1.65
Fresh Cream Fruited Scones	X 2	360	7.9	48.1	1.50
Fresh Cream Strawberry Custard Tarts	X 2	264	8.0	28.5	1.50
Fresh Cream Jam Doughnuts	X 2	260	8.6	25.2	1.65
Lemon & Raspberry Cheesecake	X 2	332	10.6	34.4	2.50
Mango & Passion Fruit Cheesecake	6 "	345	11.4	35.5	4.00
Fresh Cream Slices	X 2	354	11.9	32.5	1.65
Raspberry Cheesecake	X 2	357	12.3	19.4	2.00
Chocolate Salted Caramel Cheesecake	X 2	389	13.5	39.5	2.50
Belgian Chocolate Cheesecake	6 "	412	14.5	39.4	4.00

VALUES SHOWN PER CAKE OR 1/6TH SLICE OF A WHOLE CAKE

Cereals for Breakfast

(Excludes Breakfast Bars)

Suggested Brands	Size (g)	Kcal	S.fat (g)	Carbs (g)	£
General Mills Lucky Charms Frosted Toasted Oat Cereal with Marshmallows	422	244.2	0	48.6	5.00
Kellogg's Frosties	750	225	0.06	52.2	2.89
Kellogg's Corn Flakes Big Pack	1000	226.8	0.12	50.4	3.00
Sainsbury's Balance Cereal	500	229.2	0.12	50.88	1.25
Tesco Blueberry Wheats Cereal	500	199.8	0.18	42.48	1.80
Sainsbury's Wholegrain Blueberry Wheats	500	199.8	0.18	42.48	1.80
essential Waitrose Blueberry Wheats	500	199.8	0.18	42.48	2.05
Tesco Apricot Wheats	500	201	0.18	42.78	1.80
Sainsbury's Wholegrain Apricot Wheats	500	201	0.18	42.78	1.80
Morrisons Mini Apricot Neat Wheats	500	201	0.18	42.78	1.90
essential Waitrose wholegrain apricot wheats	500	201	0.18	42.78	2.05
Tesco Raisin Wheats	500	204	0.18	42.72	1.80
ASDA Sultana Bran	550	210.6	0.18	40.2	1.49
Stockwell & Co 24 Wheat Biscuits	432	211.2	0.18	40.44	0.75
Honey Monster Wheat Puffs Cereal	520	214.2	0.18	44.4	2.90
Morrisons Mighty Malties	625	220.8	0.18	43.8	1.25

Suggested Brands	Size (g)	Kcal	S.fat (g)	Carbs (g)	£
Tesco Low Fat Special Flake Cereal	500	222	0.18	48.6	1.25
Kellogg's Just Right Cereal	500	222.6	0.18	47.4	3.14
Kellogg's Special K Original	750	225	0.18	47.4	3.00
Kellogg's Special K Red Berries Cereal	360	225.6	0.18	47.4	2.98
ASDA Special Flakes	500	228	0.18	50.4	1.04
Waitrose LoveLife Calorie Controlled special choice rice & wheat flakes	500	228	0.18	50.4	1.99
Sainsbury's Balance With Red Fruit	375	229.8	0.18	49.74	1.25
Tesco Cornflakes	500	231.6	0.18	51.06	0.60
Morrisons Cornflakes	500	231.6	0.18	51.06	1.00
essential Waitrose corn flakes	500	231.6	0.18	51.06	1.05
ASDA Frosted Flakes	500	232.2	0.18	52.8	0.98
Tesco Frosted Flakes	500	232.2	0.18	52.8	1.00
Morrisons Frosted Flakes	500	232.2	0.18	52.8	1.25
Sainsbury's Rice Pops	500	236.4	0.18	53.1	1.50
Morrisons Sultana Bran	500	211.8	0.24	40.8	1.50
Tesco Bran Flakes	750	213.6	0.24	38.58	1.04
Kellogg's Bran Flakes	375	215.4	0.24	39	1.25
Sainsbury's Wholegrain Malties Cereal	750	219.6	0.24	43.08	1.30
Tesco Strawberry Milkshake Malt Wheats	375	221.4	0.24	43.14	1.30
ASDA Right Start	500	222	0.24	47.4	1.45
Tesco Special Flake Fruit	375	222	0.24	47.94	1.50
Morrisons Right Balance	500	222	0.24	47.28	1.58

Suggested Brands	Size (g)	Kcal	S.fat (g)	Carbs (g)	£
Sainsbury's Multigrain Hoops	375	224.4	0.24	44.64	1.20
Tesco Malt Wheats	750	226.8	0.24	45.18	1.00
ASDA Rice Snaps	340	231	0.24	51	0.98
Tesco Rice Snaps	375	231	0.24	51.06	1.00
Morrisons Rice Crackles	440	231	0.24	51.06	1.25
essential Waitrose rice pops	440	231	0.24	51.06	1.39
Dorset Cereals Simply Fruity Muesli	820	201.6	0.3	40.8	3.70
Tesco 50% Fruit Muesli	750	204	0.3	41.52	2.00
essential Waitrose sultana bran	750	206.4	0.3	39.36	1.89
ASDA Bran Flakes	500	216	0.3	38.4	0.99
Morrisons Bran Flakes	625	216	0.3	38.4	1.37
Nestle Shredded Wheat Cereal	X 30	216	0.3	40.2	2.00
Shredded Wheat Bitesize	500	220.2	0.3	41.4	2.70
Morrisons Super Hoops	375	229.2	0.3	45	1.25
Tesco Multigrain Hoops	375	229.2	0.3	45	1.50
ASDA High Bran	500	201	0.36	30	1.19
Morrisons Fantastic High Fibre	500	204.6	0.36	30.96	1.27
Sainsbury's Wholewheat Biscuits, Cereal x24	430	214.8	0.36	40.86	1.40
Essential Waitrose - Wholewheat Biscuits	X 24	214.8	0.36	40.8	1.45
ASDA Wheat Bisks	24 pack	214.8	0.36	40.8	1.59
Tesco Wheat Biscuits 24 pack	24 pack	214.8	0.36	40.8	1.60

Suggested Brands	Size (g)	Kcal	S.fat (g)	Carbs (g)	£
Morrisons Wheat Biscuits	48 pack	214.8	0.36	40.8	2.64
Sainsbury's Wholewheat Biscuits Cereal, Basics x24	432	215.4	0.36	41.1	0.80
essential Waitrose bran flakes	750	215.4	0.36	39.78	1.37
Weetabix Biscuits	72 pack	217.2	0.36	41.4	5.00
Sainsbury's Wholegrain Bran Flakes	1000	217.8	0.36	40.26	1.30
Kellogg's Frosted Wheats	600	218.4	0.36	43.2	3.00
Nestle Nesquik Cereal	375	221.4	0.36	45.6	2.00
Nestle Coco Shreddies	500	222.6	0.36	45	1.30
Kellogg's Toy Story Multigrain Shapes Cereal	350	229.8	0.36	46.8	2.00
Sainsbury's Cornflakes	500	231.6	0.36	50.34	1.00
Kellogg's All-Bran Original	500	200.4	0.42	28.8	2.40
Morrisons Choco Hoops	375	222.6	0.42	45	1.25
Nestle Honey Cheerios	565	226.8	0.42	44.4	2.00
Nestle Cookie Crisp	500	232.8	0.42	45.6	2.85
Tesco Crunchy Cookie Cereal	325	233.4	0.42	45.96	1.30
Kellogg's Crunchy Nut Original Cereal	300	237.6	0.42	49.2	1.99
Kellogg's Crunchy Nut Corn Flakes Cereal	720	238.8	0.42	49.2	3.00
Tesco High Fibre Bran	750	210	0.48	32.4	1.45
Weetabix Crunchy Bran	375	210.6	0.48	32.4	2.38
Mornflake Original Heart Healthy Oatbran Flakes	500	225.6	0.48	39.9	2.00

Suggested Brands	Size (g)	Kcal	S.fat (g)	Carbs (g)	£
Alpen no added sugar muesli	1000	221.4	0.54	37.8	4.00
Tesco No Added Sugar Swiss Style Muesli	1000	222	0.54	39.36	2.20
Alpen Original Muesli	750	224.4	0.54	39.6	2.00
Alpen original	750	224.4	0.54	39.6	2.95
ASDA Apple & Blueberry Porridge Oats	288	228	0.54	41.4	0.89
Nestle Cheerios	600	228	0.54	43.2	3.30
Kellogg's Coco Pops	480	229.2	0.54	50.4	2.89
ASDA Smart Price Porridge Oats	1000	219	0.6	38.4	0.75
ASDA Scottish Porridge Oats	1000	220.2	0.6	36.6	0.89
ASDA British Porridge Oats	500	221.4	0.6	36.6	0.74
ASDA Free From Pure Porridge Oats	450	222.6	0.6	37.2	1.79
Quaker Oat So Simple Golden Syrup Porridge	360	238.8	0.6	42.6	2.74
Nature's Path Organic Millet Rice	375	240	0.6	43.8	3.39
Tesco Honey Nut	500	241.8	0.6	49.32	1.00
Morrisons Honey Nut Corn Flakes	500	241.8	0.6	49.32	1.50
Quaker Oats So Simple Protein Original Porridge	308	228	0.66	31.8	2.75
Nestle Curiously Cinnamon	565	252	0.66	45	1.77
Essential Waitrose - Fruit Muesli	1000	206.4	0.72	39.96	2.50

Suggested Brands	Size (g)	Kcal	S.fat (g)	Carbs (g)	£
Jordans Chunky Traditional Porridge Oats	750	214.8	0.72	38.16	1.98
Waitrose Free From Gluten Free Rolled Porridge Oats	1000	221.4	0.72	34.92	4.00
ASDA Ready Oats	750	224.4	0.72	34.8	1.27
ASDA Ready Oats	750	224.4	0.72	34.8	1.27
Weetabix Ready Brek Super Smooth Original Porridge	450	224.4	0.72	34.8	1.98
Weetabix Ready Brek Super Smooth Original Porridge	180	224.4	0.72	34.8	1.98
Ready Brek Caramel Flavour Smooth Porridge Oats Sachets	180	225	0.72	38.4	1.98
Kellogg's All-Bran Golden Crunch	390	244.2	0.72	37.8	2.88
Essential Waitrose - Porridge Oats	1000	220.2	0.78	33.66	1.39
Mornflake Mighty Oats Organic Porridge Oats	1000	220.2	0.78	33.66	2.00
Waitrose Duchy Organic rolled jumbo oats	1000	220.2	0.78	33.66	2.25
Mornflake Creamy Superfast Oats	2000	220.2	0.78	33.66	2.35
Quaker Oat So Simple Original Porridge	324	222	0.78	35.4	2.74
Dorset Simply Nutty	700	231	0.78	35.88	3.70
Nestle Almond Oats & More	425	242.4	0.78	40.2	2.00

Suggested Brands	Size (g)	Kcal	S.fat (g)	Carbs (g)	£
Morrisons Oat Malties	500	244.2	0.78	35.4	1.50
Nestle Lion Cereal	400	245.4	0.78	45.6	2.00
ASDA Oatbran & Wheatbran Porridge Oats	500	223.2	0.84	34.8	0.59
Nestle Oat Cheerios Low Sugar	325	239.4	0.84	39.6	2.50
Quaker Porridge Oats	1000	224.4	0.9	36	1.98
Scott's Porage Original Scottish Porridge Oats	1000	224.4	0.9	36	2.00
Quaker Porridge Jumbo Oats	1000	224.4	0.9	36	2.18
Scott's Porage Old Fashioned Porridge Oats	1000	224.4	0.9	36	2.28
Tesco Choco Snaps	350	233.4	0.9	50.16	1.00
Morrisons Choco Crackles	440	233.4	0.9	50.16	1.25
ASDA Choco Snaps	550	233.4	0.9	50.4	1.59
essential Waitrose Choco Pops	550	237	0.9	51.06	1.60
Nestle Cheerios Oat Cereal	379	237	0.9	42	2.99
ASDA Coconut Flavour Porridge Oats Sachets	288	225	0.96	39	0.89
Kellogg's White Choc Coco Pops Cereal	480	231	0.96	48.6	2.00
Mornflake Mighty Oats Original Heart Healthy Oatbran	800	218.4	1.08	28.38	2.00
Ready Brek Chocolate Smooth Porridge	192	225.6	1.08	37.2	1.98
Tesco Honey Nut Clusters	500	264.6	1.08	39.42	1.50
ASDA Chocolate Flavour Ready Oats	450	229.2	1.32	38.4	1.25

Suggested Brands	Size (g)	Kcal	S.fat (g)	Carbs (g)	£
Weetabix Ready Brek Super Smooth Chocolate Porridge	450	229.2	1.32	38.4	1.98
White's Wild Fruit Crunch Toasted Oats	500	265.8	1.32	40.2	2.00
Jordans Raisin & Almond Nut Granola	750	247.2	1.38	36.96	2.00
Mornflake Chocolately Squares	375	268.8	1.86	42.06	1.00
Lizi's High Protein Granola	350	270	1.86	26.4	3.00
Jordans Country Crisp Delicious Honey & Nut	500	269.4	1.92	37.62	3.00
Sainsbury's Wholegrain Fruit & Fibre	1000	223.2	1.98	39.66	1.95
Waitrose Honey Raisin & Almond Oat Crunchy	1000	246.6	1.98	37.86	2.30
Kellogg's Fruit 'n Fibre	750	228	2.1	41.4	2.97
Essential Waitrose - Fruit & Nut Muesli	1000	231.6	2.22	34.5	2.50
Tesco Pillows With Milk Chocolate Filling	375	273.6	2.28	41.1	1.10
Tesco Pillows Chocolate Nut	375	277.8	2.34	39.42	1.10
Kellogg's Krave Chocolate	375	264.6	2.4	42	2.00
essential Waitrose fruit & fibre	750	229.8	2.46	41.1	1.89
Lizi's Low Sugar Granola	500	300.6	2.52	27.12	2.30
ASDA Fruit & Fibre	750	232.2	2.58	41.4	1.45
Morrisons Fruit & Fibre	500	232.2	2.58	41.4	3.00
Tesco Honey Nut Chocolate Clusters	500	272.4	2.58	38.58	1.50

Suggested Brands	Size (g)	Kcal	S.fat (g)	Carbs (g)	£
Jordans Crunchy Oat Granola Fruit & Nut	750	256.2	2.64	38.52	2.00
Tesco Fruit Nut Muesli	750	231.6	2.94	36.06	2.00
Morrisons The Best Nut & Seed Granola	500	289.2	4.2	33.3	2.30
Waitrose Seriously chocolatey triple chocolate crisp	500	270	4.26	37.86	2.15
Kellogg's Crunchy Nut Glorious Oat Granola Cracking	600	298.2	7.2	34.2	3.20

VALUES SHOWN PER 60 GRAM SERVING

Your Favourite Food Not Included?
Let Us Know

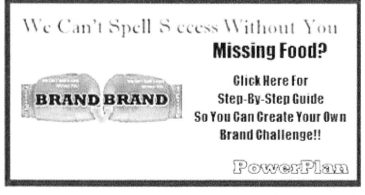
WWW.WECANTSPELLSUCCESSWITHOUTYOU.COM

Cheese

Suggested Brands	Size (g)	Kcal	S.fat (g)	Carbs (g)	£
Tesco Quark Fat Free Soft Cheese	250	63	0	3.5	0.90
Grahams Quark Fat Free Soft Cheese	250	65	0.05	3.7	1.00
E ssential Waitrose Fat Free Quark Soft Cheese	250	71	0.05	5.1	0.90
Sainsbury's Cottage Cheese, Fat Free	300	74	0.06	7.4	1.40
Iceland Cottage Cheese	250	57	0.2	3.0	0.70
ASDA Fat Free Cottage Cheese	300	62	0.3	4.7	1.00
Tesco Fat Free Cottage Cheese	300	62	0.3	4.7	1.00
Morrisons Savers Cottage Cheese	300	69	0.5	3.3	0.64
The Laughing Cow Extra Light Cheese Triangles	140	116	1.3	11	1.40
Philadelphia Lightest Soft Cheese	180	90	1.7	5.5	1.00
Sainsbury's Cottage Cheese	300	107	3.3	3.8	1.40
essential Waitrose natural cottage cheese	300	105	3.8	4.2	1.30
The Laughing Cow Light Cheese Triangles	280	147	4.7	6	2.00
Dairylea Cheese Spread	270	201	4.8	9.2	1.50
Apetina Light Cheese	200	173	6.4	0.6	1.50
Morrisons 45% Lighter Italian Mozarella	125	173	7	2.1	0.65

Suggested Brands	Size (g)	Kcal	S.fat (g)	Carbs (g)	£
Weight Watchers Grated Mature Cheddar	200	214	7.1	4.3	2.00
Weight Watchers 8 Mature Cheese Slices	160	232	7.1	3.5	2.00
Sainsbury's Lighter Mozzarella Cheese, Be Good To Yourself	125	172	7.2	0.05	0.70
Philadelphia Light Soft Cheese	180	150	7.4	5.2	1.00
Tesco 50% Less Fat Soft Cheese	200	161	7.6	5.4	0.80
essential Waitrose reduced fat soft cheese	250	161	7.6	5.4	1.10
Dairylea 8 Cheese Slices	200	223	8.4	8.8	1.00
Dairylea Cheese Triangles x8	125	208	9.8	4.7	1.18
Waitrose essential Italian Mozzarella	125	213	10.6	0.4	0.70
Creamfields 10 Cheesy Slices	170	278	10.9	7.6	0.59
ASDA 50% Less Fat Mature Cheese	500	287	11	0.05	2.49
Morrisons Halloumi	225	270	11.7	1.6	2.20
Creamfields Mozzarella	125	234	12	1.0	0.45
Creamfields Mozzarella	125	234	12	1.0	0.45
Sainsbury's Italian Mozzarella Cheese	150	222	12.1	1.7	0.75
The Laughing Cow Original Cheese Triangles	280	239	12.5	6.5	2.00
Tesco Mozzarella	150	230	12.7	0.6	0.70

COMMON FOOD   CHEESE

Suggested Brands	Size (g)	Kcal	S.fat (g)	Carbs (g)	£
Sainsbury's Mozzarella Cheese, Basics	125	245	13	1.5	0.50
ASDA Grated Mozzarella Cheese	250	295	13	2.4	1.90
ASDA 10 Mozzarella Cheese Slices	220	295	13	2.4	1.90
Sainsbury's Cypriot Light Halloumi Cheese	225	277	13.1	2.6	2.30
Iceland Mozzarella	250	285	13.2	2.1	2.00
Creamfields Lighter Mature Cheese	400	314	13.8	0.8	1.79
Tesco Cheddar 30% Less Fat	460	314	13.8	0.8	2.30
Pilgrims Choice Lighter Mature Cheese	350	314	13.8	0.8	3.50
Philadelphia Original Soft Cheese	180	225	14	4.3	1.00
Iceland Greek Feta Cheese	200	252	14	1.3	1.35
Apetina Classic Block Cheese	200	274	14	0.03	1.50
Sainsbury's Somerset Brie Cheese	160	291	14.6	0.05	1.50
Waitrose mild Somerset Brie cheese	230	291	14.6	0.05	2.10
Morrisons 45% Lighter Italian Mozarella	200	307	14.6	5.1	1.40
Morrisons Cheddar 30% Less Fat	250	324	14.6	3	1.90
essential Waitrose 30% Lighter Extra Mature Chees	350	337	14.6	3.0	3.00

Suggested Brands	Size (g)	Kcal	S.fat (g)	Carbs (g)	£
Creamfields Greek Style Salad Cheese	299	266	14.7	1.9	0.75
Waitrose creamy & tangy Greek feta	200	283	15	0.2	1.99
Tesco French Ripening Brie	190	275	15.1	1.1	1.80
Pilgrims Choice Lighter Extra Mature Cheddar	350	323	15.1	0.2	3.50
Sainsbury's Soft Cheese, Basics	300	202	15.6	3.3	0.75
Creamfields Soft Cheese	200	239	15.6	4.7	0.49
Iceland Halloumi	250	303	15.8	2.3	2.00
ASDA Smart Price Soft Cheese	300	239	16	4.7	0.74
ASDA Grated Four Cheese Blend	200	333	16	2.7	1.90
ASDA 30% Less Fat Mild Cheddar Cheese	500	337	16	0.05	2.49
Cathedral City Kids Snack Nibbles	30	331	16.4	0.1	1.50
Cathedral City Mature Lighter Cheese	350	331	16.4	0.1	3.50
Morrisons Greek Feta	200	281	16.7	3.1	1.35
Iceland Mellow & Buttery Somerset Brie	150	306	16.8	1.3	1.40
Morrisons British Somerset Brie	160	302	16.9	1.9	1.56
Sainsburys Greek Cheese Feta	200	276	17	0.7	1.35
essential Waitrose Greek Feta cheese	200	276	17	0.7	1.45

Suggested Brands	Size (g)	Kcal	S.fat (g)	Carbs (g)	£
Sainsbury's Feta Cheese, SO Organic	200	276	17	0.7	2.00
ASDA Feta Cheese	200	278	17	0.7	1.05
Mlekovita Ser Gouda Slices	150	334	17	0	1.06
Dairylea Strip Cheese x8	168	336	17	3.5	2.00
Tesco Greek Cheese Feta	200	279	17.1	1.0	1.20
Waitrose Duchy Organic Feta cheese,	200	289	17.7	0.1	2.50
Creamfields Grana Padano	200	398	18	0	1.89
Sainsbury's Cypriot Halloumi Cheese	225	328	18.2	0.9	2.30
essential Waitrose Cypriot halloumi cheese	250	328	18.2	0.9	2.55
Yamas Chilli Halloumi Cheese	225	353	18.2	1.2	2.60
Morrisons The Best Halloum	225	336	18.3	2.2	3.00
Sainsbury's Soft Cheese, SO Organic	250	253	18.4	3.1	1.50
Waitrose Duchy Organic soft cheese	250	281	18.4	3.7	1.85
Morrisons Extra Mature 10 Cheddar Slices	250	402	18.7	3	2.00
Sainsbury's Soft White Cheese	300	255	19	3.1	1.20
Morrisons Soft Cheese Full Fat	250	279	19	3.1	1.00
ASDA Creamy Original Soft Cheese	200	285	19	4.0	0.69

Suggested Brands	Size (g)	Kcal	S.fat (g)	Carbs (g)	£
Tesco Soft Cheese Plain Full Fat	200	285	19	4.0	0.80
essential Waitrose creamy soft cheese, strength	250	285	19	4.0	1.10
Tesco Halloumi	225	336	19.3	2.2	2.00
Morrisons Red Leicester Cheese	400	401	19.3	3.4	2.50
Morrisons Cheddar Mature	400	295	19.4	2.3	2.50
Morrisons Cheddar mild	400	405	20.2	3.4	2.50
ASDA Cheshire Cheese	250	386	21	0.3	1.75
ASDA Red Leicester Cheese	500	403	21	0.05	2.49
ASDA Smart Price Red Leicester	825	403	21	0.05	3.49
Sainsbury's Red Leicester Cheese, SO Organic	270	399	21.1	0.0	2.50
Tesco Red Leicester Cheese	220	403	21.1	0.1	1.55
Sainsburys Red Leicester Cheese	250	403	21.1	0.05	1.75
Creamfields Red Leicester Cheese	400	403	21.1	0.05	1.79
Iceland Red Leicester Cheese	250	403	21.1	0.1	2.00
essential Waitrose medium Red Leicester cheese, strength	350	411	21.6	0.05	2.60
Waitrose Somerset Cheddar Mature Strength	350	410	21.7	0.05	4.00

Suggested Brands	Size (g)	Kcal	S.fat (g)	Carbs (g)	£
Sainsbury's British Mature Cheddar Cheese Slices	240	416	21.7	0.05	1.70
Creamfields Mild White Cheddar Large	400	416	21.7	0.1	1.79
Creamfields Mature White Cheddar Large	400	416	21.7	0.1	1.79
Creamfields Medium White Cheddar	400	416	21.7	0.1	1.79
essential Waitrose English medium Cheddar cheese, strength 3, 10 slices	250	416	21.7	0.05	1.89
Morrisons Organic Mature Cheddar	250	416	21.7	0.0	1.90
Tesco Mature 10 Cheddar Slices	250	416	21.7	0.1	1.90
Sainsbury's British Mature Cheddar Cheese	400	416	21.7	0.05	2.00
Sainsbury's British Mild Cheddar Cheese	400	416	21.7	0.05	2.00
Cathedral City 8 Mature Cheddar Cheese Slices	150	416	21.7	0.1	2.00
Iceland Mature 10 Cheddar Slices	250	416	21.7	0.1	2.00
Tesco Cheddar mild	460	416	21.7	0.1	2.30
Sainsbury's Mature Cheddar Cheese, SO Organic	270	416	21.7	0.05	2.50
Sainsbury's Mild Cheddar Cheese, SO Organic	270	416	21.7	0.05	2.50
essential Waitrose English Mild Cheddar Strength	550	416	21.7	0.05	3.00

COMMON FOOD   CHEESE

Suggested Brands	Size (g)	Kcal	S.fat (g)	Carbs (g)	£
Cathedral City Mature Cheddar Cheese	350	416	21.7	0.1	3.50
Cathedral City Extra Mature Cheddar Cheese	350	416	21.7	0.1	3.50
Pilgrims Choice Extra Mature Cheddar Cheese	350	416	21.7	0.1	3.50
Cathedral City Vintage Cheddar Cheese	300	416	21.7	0.1	3.50
Pilgrims Choice Mature Cheddar Cheese	350	416	21.7	0.1	3.50
Pilgrims Choice Vintage Cheddar Cheese	300	416	21.7	0.1	3.50
Waitrose Duchy Organic extra mature Cheddar	350	416	21.7	0.05	3.85
Iceland Cheddar Mature	800	416	21.7	0.1	3.85
Iceland Cheddar mild	800	416	21.7	0.1	3.85
Orsom Woodew Handmade Smoked Cheddar	200	416	21.7	0.1	2.50
Creamfields French Brie	200	364	22	1.0	0.79
ASDA Double Gloucester Cheese	500	413	22	0.4	2.49
Lactofree Mature Cheddar	200	416	22	0.05	1.50
ASDA Extra Special Wyke Farms Extra Mature Cheddar	200	416	22	0.3	2.15
ASDA Smart Price Mild White Cheddar	825	416	22	0.05	3.65
ASDA Smart Price Mature White Cheddar	825	416	22	0.05	3.69

Common Food   Cheese

Suggested Brands	Size (g)	Kcal	S.fat (g)	Carbs (g)	£
ASDA 10 Mature Cheddar Cheese Slices	250	417	22	0.05	1.90
ASDA Mature Cheddar Cheese	500	417	22	0.05	2.49
ASDA Mild Cheddar Cheese	500	417	22	0.05	2.49
ASDA Extra Mature Cheddar Cheese	500	417	22	0.05	2.49
ASDA Medium Cheddar Cheese	500	417	22	0.05	2.49
Red Fox Aged Red Leicester	200	425	22.4	2.7	2.50
essential Waitrose French mild Brie cheese	200	356	23	0.0	1.60
Creamfields Halloumi	225	313	24.6	0.8	1.39
Tesco Cheddar Mature	460	416	34.9	0.1	2.30

Values Shown Per 100 Grams

Find Us On

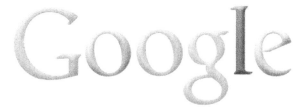

Search: **NADIET.INFO**

Chips

Suggested Brands	Size (g)	Kcal	S.fat (g)	Carbs (g)	£
Home Air/Acti-Fry Organic Chips with 1 cal oil spray	1500	204.5	0.3	42.3	2.00
Slimming World Free Food Chips	1000	295.4	0.3	59.4	2.25
Home Air/Acti-Fry Organic Chips with 15ml oil	1500	312.4	0.3	42.3	2.00
ASDA Straight Cut Chips less than 3% oven baked	1500	380.6	0.9	68.2	1.25
Iceland Low Fat Straight Cut Chips	1200	394.8	0.9	71.6	1.00
Waitrose Frozen Crisp & Fluffy Chunky Chips	1000	400.4	0.9	71.9	1.69
McCain Lighter Home Chips Straight	1360	403.3	0.9	73.8	2.30
Sainsbury's Straight Cut Oven Chips, Be Good To Yourself	900	428.8	0.9	78.7	1.20
Morrisons Eat Smart Oven Chips	900	451.6	0.9	83.5	1.00
Tesco Finest Chunky Chips With Sea Salt	450	474.3	0.9	84.1	2.60
Aunt Bessie's Crispy & Fluffy Homestyle Chips	600	329.4	1.1	51.1	0.79
McCain Original Oven Chips 5% Fat Straight Cut	1360	374.9	1.1	63.3	2.15
Sainsbury's Super Chunky Chips	900	411.8	1.1	68.2	1.15

Suggested Brands	Size (g)	Kcal	S.fat (g)	Carbs (g)	£
Aunt Bessie's Deliciously Crisp French Fries	700	426.0	1.1	73.8	1.00
Waitrose chunky chips	450	448.7	1.1	75.3	2.19
Sainsbury's Chunky Maris Piper Chips, Taste the Difference	1500	477.1	1.1	82.6	2.40
essential Waitrose steak cut oven chips	900	380.6	1.4	62.8	1.25
McCain Home Chips Straight	1360	409.0	1.4	65.3	2.30
Iceland Steak Cut Chips	1250	443.0	1.4	69.9	1.00
McCain Quick Chips Straight x 6 100g	600	445.9	1.4	75.0	2.00
Iceland Crinkle Cut Chips	1250	457.2	1.4	76.4	1.00
Iceland Straight Cut Chips	1250	465.8	1.4	73.8	1.00
ASDA Extra Special Chunky Maris Piper Chips	750	480.0	1.4	88.0	1.95
Tesco Oven Chips	450	485.6	1.4	70.7	2.25
Morrisons Free From Homestyle Chips	750	494.2	1.4	87.8	1.00
Tesco Homestyle Straight Cut Oven Chips	950	494.2	1.4	87.8	1.35
Tesco Homestyle Crinkle Cut Oven Chips	950	502.7	1.4	86.6	1.35
Iceland Ridiculously Crispy Crinkle Cut Chips	1200	502.7	1.4	81.2	1.50
Morrisons The Best Chunky Chips	1500	502.7	1.4	89.2	2.50
McCain Crispy Sweet Potato Fries	500	355.0	1.7	41.2	2.50

COMMON FOOD   CHIPS

Suggested Brands	Size (g)	Kcal	S.fat (g)	Carbs (g)	£
Tesco Salt & Pepper Ridge Chips	750	454.4	1.7	69.9	1.50
Albert Bartlett Rooster Deep Crinkle Cut Chips	1200	471.4	1.7	65.3	2.50
Morrisons The Best Maris Piper Chunky Chips	450	485.6	1.7	80.1	2.00
ASDA Seasoned Sweet Potato Fries	500	497.0	1.7	73.8	1.98
Tesco Sweet Potato Oven Chips	500	497.0	1.7	74.4	2.30
Disney Kitchen French Fries	1000	499.8	1.7	78.4	1.00
Morrisons Crinkle Cut Chips	2000	508.4	1.7	78.7	1.80
Iceland Alphabet Potato Shapes	550	519.7	1.7	82.9	1.00
Iceland Luxury Maris Piper Chunky Oven Chips	1500	551.0	1.7	94.3	2.00
ASDA Homestyle Chips	1500	565.2	1.7	90.9	1.90
McCain Home Chips Crinkle	1360	414.6	2.0	56.8	2.30
Waitrose sweet potato oven chips	500	440.2	2.0	56.5	2.45
Morrisons Steak Cut Chips	1200	451.6	2.0	70.1	1.20
Disney Kitchen Olaf Potato Shapes	500	502.7	2.0	76.7	1.00
ASDA Smart Price Chips	1500	528.2	2.0	82.4	0.90
Morrisons Straight Cut Chips	1200	528.2	2.0	82.4	1.20

Suggested Brands	Size (g)	Kcal	S.fat (g)	Carbs (g)	£
Sainsbury's Seasoned Rustic Fries	900	528.2	2.0	81.5	1.25
ASDA Straight Cut Chips	1500	528.2	2.0	82.4	1.25
Sainsbury's Straight Cut Chips	1500	528.2	2.0	82.4	1.50
Tesco Curly Fries	700	536.8	2.0	84.1	1.50
Tesco Finest British Chunky Oven Chips	1500	545.3	2.0	99.7	2.50
Sainsbury's French Fries	900	610.6	2.0	102.2	1.20
Iceland Thin & Crispy French Fries	1250	622.0	2.0	100.0	1.00
ASDA French Fries	1500	644.7	2.0	105.1	1.25
Tesco French Fries	1500	710.0	2.0	117.0	1.25
Sainsbury's Steak Cut Chips	1500	409.0	2.3	71.0	1.50
McCain Our Menu Signatures Smiles	907	502.7	2.3	73.6	2.00
McCain Crispy French Fries	1200	522.6	2.3	76.4	2.60
Sainsbury's Lightly Spiced Fries	900	573.7	2.3	88.0	1.25
Iceland Ridiculously Crispy Straight Cut Chips	1200	596.4	2.3	89.5	1.50
Sainsbury's Crinkle Cut Chips	900	471.4	2.6	76.7	1.20
ASDA Crinkle Cut Chips	1500	474.3	2.6	76.7	1.25
Sainsbury's Chips, Basics	900	536.8	2.6	84.9	0.80
McCain Spicy Peri Peri Fries	650	553.8	2.6	72.4	2.50
Tesco Crispy Sweet Potato Fries	300	604.9	2.6	61.3	2.50

Common Food   Chips

Suggested Brands	Size (g)	Kcal	S.fat (g)	Carbs (g)	£
Iceland Curly Fries	750	1048.0	2.6	112.2	1.50
Tesco Crinkle Cut Oven Chips	1500	460.1	2.8	75.8	1.25
Tesco Steak Oven Cut Chips	1500	460.1	2.8	75.8	1.25
McCain Quick Cook Crispy French Fries	750	630.5	2.8	89.7	2.75
Sainsbury's Seasoned Curly Fries	700	727.0	2.8	101.1	1.50
Iceland Sweet Potato Fries	600	565.2	3.1	63.6	2.00
ASDA Curly Fries	750	641.8	3.7	79.5	1.15
Iceland Criss Cross Fries	700	735.6	4.0	95.7	1.50
Iceland Southern Fried Chips	850	769.6	4.0	92.6	1.50
Sainsbury's Sweet Potato Fries	500	536.8	4.5	85.5	2.30
Straight Cut Value Fry Chips	1500	397.6	5.7	61.6	1.00
essential Waitrose French Fries	900	417.5	7.1	64.2	1.25
McCain Triple Cooked Gastro Chips	640	576.5	8.5	59.6	2.50
Iceland Ridiculously Chunky Skin On Chips	900	619.1	12.2	61.3	1.50
Sainsbury's Triple Cooked Chips, Taste the Difference	900	596.4	12.8	79.0	2.25
Fries to Go Original X 2 90g	180	698.6	20.7	114.2	1.00

COMMON FOOD CHIPS

Suggested Brands	Size (g)	Kcal	S.fat (g)	Carbs (g)	£
Tesco Skin On Chunky Chips	500	235.7	25.8	46.6	1.00
Halloumi Fries	190	925.8	46.6	5.1	3.00

VALUES SHOWN PER 284 GRAMS SERVING

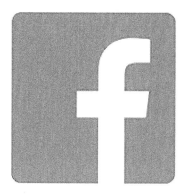

www.facebook.com/StephendDBarnes

Cooking Oil

Suggested Brands	Size (g)	Kcal	S.fat (g)	Carbs (g)	£
ASDA Extra Special Cold-Pressed Rapeseed Oil	500	124	0.9	0.0	1.59
Sainsbury's Rapeseed Oil, SO Organic	1000	124	0.9	0.0	3.60
Tesco Pure Vegetable Oil	1000	135	1.0	0.0	1.20
Asda Vegetable Oil	1000	124	1.1	0.0	1.09
Goldenfields Pure Rapeseed Oil	1000	124	1.1	0.0	1.70
Mazola Pure Rapeseed Oil	1000	124	1.1	0.0	2.00
Crisp N Dry	2000	124	1.1	0.0	3.50
Olivio Oil	500	124	1.2	0.0	1.50
ASDA Sunflower Oil	1000	124	1.5	0.0	1.09
ASDA Sunflower Oil	1000	124	1.5	0.0	1.09
Morrisons Vegetable Oil	1000	124	1.5	0.0	1.15
ASDA Grapeseed Oil	500	124	1.5	0.0	2.75
Sainsbury's Stir Fry Oil	250	124	1.6	0.0	1.60
Sainsbury's Grapeseed Oil	500	125	1.6	0.0	2.75
Morrisons Sunflower Oil	1000	124	1.7	0.0	1.15
Tesco Pure Sunflower Oil	1000	135	1.7	0.0	1.20
Mazola Pure Corn Oil	1000	124	1.9	0.0	2.34
KTC Pure Corn Oil	1000	135	1.9	0.0	2.00
ASDA Olive Oil	1000	123	2.0	0.0	2.98
ASDA Extra Virgin Olive Oil	1000	123	2.0	0.0	3.40
ASDA Sesame Seed Oil	250	124	2.0	0.0	1.39
Sainsbury's Corn Oil	1000	124	2.0	0.0	1.75
Carotino Healthier Oil	500	124	2.1	0.0	2.00
Carotino Mild & Light Cooking	500	124	2.1	0.0	2.00

COMMON FOOD COOKING OIL

Suggested Brands	Size (g)	Kcal	S.fat (g)	Carbs (g)	£
KTC 100% Pure Coconut Cooking Oil	650	135	12.8	0.0	2.50

VALUES SHOWN PER 15 ML SERVING

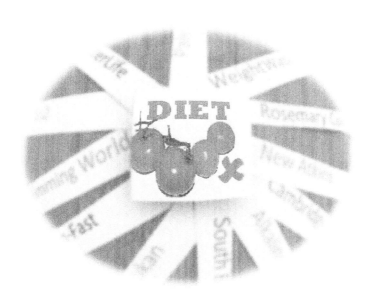

Cous Cous

Suggested Brands	Size (g)	Kcal	S.fat (g)	Carbs (g)	£
Morrisons Wholefoods	500	54	0.0	10.9	0.70
Waitrose Cauliflower & Kale	300	72	0.0	9.9	2.00
Gefen Israeli	250	81	0.0	37.8	1.00
Ella's Kitchen Veggie	120	23	0.1	3.9	1.50
Waitrose LoveLife Calorie Controlled roasted vegetable	280	50	0.1	9.0	2.50
essential Waitrose	500	56	0.1	11.6	0.68
Iceland 4 Vegetable Couscous Steam Bags	500	57	0.1	9.3	2.00
Tesco Whole Wheat	500	60	0.1	11.1	0.70
Ainsley Harriott Sundried Tomato & Garlic	100	67	0.1	12.6	0.50
Ainsley Harriott Lemon Parsley & Mint	100	67	0.1	12.6	0.50
Ainsley Harriott Wild Mushroom	100	67	0.1	12.7	0.50
Ainsley Harriott Tomato & Chilli	100	68	0.1	12.7	0.50
Batchelors Spice Sensation	90	68	0.1	13.2	0.50
Batchelors Cous Cous Peri-Peri	90	68	0.1	13.3	0.50
Batchelors Cous Cous Chilli Beef	90	68	0.1	13.4	0.50
Ainsley Harriott Spice Sensation	100	69	0.1	12.3	0.50
Ainsley Harriott Moroccan Medley	100	69	0.1	12.6	0.50

Suggested Brands	Size (g)	Kcal	S.fat (g)	Carbs (g)	£
Ainsley Harriott Aromatic Thai Style	100	69	0.1	12.7	0.50
Batchelors Cous Cous Chicken & Roasted Vegetable	90	69	0.1	13.3	0.50
Batchelors Roasted Vegetable	90	69	0.1	13.4	0.50
Batchelors Mushroom & Garlic	90	69	0.1	13.5	0.50
Sainsbury's Cous Cous Coriander & Lemon	110	70	0.1	13.8	0.45
ASDA 2 Steam Bags Cous Cous & Quinoa Warm Salad	400	77	0.1	13.5	1.25
Waitrose Duchy Organic	500	79	0.1	15.7	1.05
Sainsbury's Cous Cous	500	81	0.1	14.9	0.70
Sainsbury's Cous Cous, SO Organic	500	81	0.1	14.9	1.20
ASDA Cous Cous	500	89	0.1	17.5	0.60
Tesco Roasted Vegetable Flavour	110	55	0.2	9.3	0.45
Sainsbury's Sundried Tomato & Garlic	110	60	0.2	11.3	0.45
ASDA Spicy Vegetable Cous Cous	500	66	0.2	9.0	1.79
ASDA Spicy Vegetable	500	66	0.2	9.0	1.79
Waitrose Roasted Vegetable	200	68	0.2	9.3	2.00
ASDA Spicy Vegetable	110	72	0.2	13.5	0.42
Morrison Spicy Vegetable	110	72	0.2	13.4	0.60

COMMON FOOD   COUS COUS

Suggested Brands	Size (g)	Kcal	S.fat (g)	Carbs (g)	£
Morrisons Tomato & Garlic	110	72	0.2	13.6	0.60
Tesco Mediterranean Style	110	73	0.2	13.4	0.45
Morrisons Mediterranean	110	73	0.2	13.9	0.60
Tesco Lemon And Coriander	110	74	0.2	13.8	0.45
GAMA	500	74	0.2	36.5	1.25
ASDA Sun-Dried Tomato	280	74	0.2	12.0	2.00
Iceland Roast Vegetable	280	75	0.2	13.0	1.00
Morrison Lemon & Coriander	110	76	0.2	14.7	0.60
Sainsbury's Chargrill Vegetable Cous Cous	200	76	0.2	13.8	1.50
ASDA Coriander & Lemon	110	78	0.2	15.0	0.42
Tesco Finest Vegetable	250	78	0.2	11.6	2.25
Waitrose LOVE life wholewheat	500	79	0.2	14.4	0.99
Morrisons Fruity	250	90	0.2	15.4	2.00
Iceland Fruity	280	91	0.2	14.8	1.00
Tesco Cous Cous	1000	102	0.2	19.1	1.35
Sainsbury's Moroccan	200	102	0.2	16.6	2.25
Gama For Goodness Sake Cous Cous	1000	175	0.2	36.5	2.05
Osem Israel	250	180	0.2	37.0	0.85
ASDA Mediterranean Style Tomato	110	74	0.3	13.0	0.42
Tesco Mushroom	110	74	0.3	13.6	0.45
Sainsbury's Roasted Vegetable	110	76	0.3	14.6	0.45
Morrisons Roasted Veg	250	80	0.3	10.2	2.00

COMMON FOOD   COUS COUS

Suggested Brands	Size (g)	Kcal	S.fat (g)	Carbs (g)	£
Morrisons Moroccan	250	98	0.3	15.7	2.25
Tesco Finest Moroccan	250	108	0.3	13.5	2.25
Cypressa Cous cous	500	177	0.3	35.0	1.00
Waitrose tomato & onion	110	73	0.4	13.2	0.93
Waitrose Moroccan Spiced Fruity	235	94	0.4	14.6	2.00
Waitrose fruity Moroccan	410	94	0.4	14.6	3.00
Ella's Kitchen 7 Mths+ Zingy Lamb Cous Cous with Apricots & Raisins	130	29	0.5	3.4	1.50
Prep Co Mediterranean Cous Cous	73	62	0.5	8.5	1.99
Waitrose lemon & garlic	110	73	0.5	13.1	0.93
Delphi Couscous With Chargrilled Vegetables And Olive Oil	160	87	0.5	13.0	1.46
Waitrose garlic & coriander	110	72	0.6	12.8	0.93
GOOD TO GO Sweet Potato, Bulgur & Couscous	290	72	0.6	7.0	3.00
Tesco Finest Toasted Cous Cous And Aged Feta	180	102	1.4	9.8	2.25

VALUES SHOWN PER 50 GRAMS

Crackers

Suggested Brands	Size (g)	Kcal	S.fat (g)	Carbs (g)	£
Schar Gluten Free Fibre Crispbread	125	22	0	4.6	1.50
Ryvita Original Crackerbread	200	19	0.02	3.8	1.35
Milton's Multigrain Crackers	170	22	0.06	3.0	1.29
Tesco Snackers	200	16	0.08	2.3	0.99
Carr's Table Water Biscuits	125	14	0.1	2.5	1.19
ASDA Cracker Bites	200	18	0.1	2.2	1.00
Ritz Cheese Crackers	200	21	0.1	2.3	1.20
Tesco Finest Assorted Cracker For Cheese	250	23	0.1	3.3	2.50
Ritz Breaks Original Crackers	190	29	0.1	4.1	1.87
Tesco High Baked Water Biscuits	200	22	0.2	4.2	0.65
ASDA Garlic Crackers	200	28	0.2	3.7	0.85
ASDA Salt & Pepper Crackers	185	29	0.2	3.7	0.79
Tesco Salt & Pepper Cracker	185	30	0.2	3.7	0.95
Tesco Poppy & Sesame Thins	150	20	0.3	2.5	0.89
ASDA Free From Plain Crackers	200	27	0.3	4.7	1.99
Marmite Biscuits For Cheese	150	29	0.3	3.9	2.00
Nairn's Gluten Free Wholegrain Crackers	137	26	0.4	3.3	1.70

COMMON FOOD CRACKERS

Suggested Brands	Size (g)	Kcal	S.fat (g)	Carbs (g)	£
Jacob's Cream Crackers High Fibre	200	34	0.4	4.5	1.19
Jacob's Choice Grain Crackers	200	32	0.5	4.7	1.19
Morrisons Cream Crackers	300	35	0.5	5.4	0.40
ASDA Cream Crackers	300	35	0.5	5.4	0.49
Sainsbury's Cream Crackers	300	35	0.5	5.4	0.50
essential Waitrose cream crackers	300	35	0.5	5.4	0.55
Jacob's Cream Crackers	200	35	0.5	5.4	1.00
Morrisons Cheese Thins	160	20	0.6	1.9	0.68
ASDA Cheese Thins	150	21	0.6	1.9	0.75
Tesco Cheese Thins	150	21	0.6	1.9	0.89
Tesco Cream Crackers	300	38	0.6	5.7	0.40
Jacob's Savours Sour Cream & Chive Thins	150	21	0.7	2.8	1.00
Carr's Cheese Melts	150	21	0.7	2.6	1.49
Tuc Original Cracker	150	26	0.7	2.7	1.00
ASDA Cracker Selection	150	36	0.7	4.7	0.95

VALUES SHOWN PER CRACKER

Crisps

Suggested Brands	Size (g)	Kcal	S.fat (g)	Carbs (g)	£
Skips	17	92	0.5	9.9	0.55
Tesco everyday salt and vinegar *	18	98	0.5	9.2	0.05
Walkers Quavers	20	107	0.5	12.0	0.55
Tesco everyday Cheese And Onion *	18	95	0.6	9.6	0.05
Tesco everyday Ready Salted *	18	96	0.6	9.5	0.05
Smart Price Ready Salted *	18	99	0.6	9.3	0.05
Walkers Smoky Bacon	25	130	0.6	13.4	0.45
Tesco Smoky Bacon *	25	87	0.7	12.6	0.13
Asda Ready Salted *	25	130	0.7	13	0.13
Asda Roast Chicken	25	130	0.7	13	0.13
Asda Cheese And Onion *	25	132	0.7	13	0.13
Morrison's smoky bacon *	25	132	0.7	13.8	0.13
Tesco salt and vinegar *	25	134	0.7	13	0.08
Tesco Roast Chicken *	25	134	0.7	12.3	0.13
Morrison's Roast chicken *	25	134	0.7	12.3	0.13
Tesco Cheese And Onion *	25	134	0.7	13	0.13
Tesco Prawn Cocktail *	25	135	0.7	12.7	0.08
Tesco Ready Salted *	25	136	0.7	13.8	0.08
Asda salt and vinegar *	25	132	0.8	13	0.13
Asda Prawn Cocktail *	25	133	0.8	13	0.13
Morrison's everyday Ready Salted *	25	136	0.8	13.1	0.13
Walkers Roast Chicken	32.5	168	0.8	17.1	0.55

Common Food   Crisps

Suggested Brands	Size (g)	Kcal	S.fat (g)	Carbs (g)	£
Walkers Cheese And Onion	32.5	169	0.8	17.1	0.55
Walkers salt and vinegar	32.5	169	0.8	17.1	0.55
Walkers Prawn Cocktail	32.5	169	0.8	17.2	0.55
Walkers Ready Salted	32.5	171	0.8	16.7	0.55

Values shown per Packet of Crisps

* Indicates Sold In The Multipack

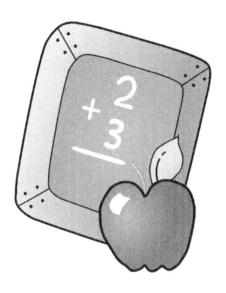

Donuts

Suggested Brands	Size (pack)	Kcal	S.fat (g)	Carbs (g)	£
ASDA Custard Donuts	2	139	2.1	20.3	1.25
Sainsbury's Custard Doughnuts	2	150	2.6	20.5	1.30
Tesco 5 Pack Jam Doughnuts	5	178	2.7	27.4	0.80
ASDA Baker's Selection Jam Donuts	5	184	2.7	29.0	0.79
Tesco Jam Doughnuts	5	193	2.7	27.3	1.00
Raspberry jam doughnut	4	179	2.9	28.2	2.00
ASDA Baker's Selection Chocolate Donut	5	184	3.0	26.7	0.79
Tesco Custard Doughnut	2	157	3.2	20.4	1.40
Custard Doughnuts	5	165	3.2	22.9	0.80
ASDA Baker's Selection Custard Donuts	5	173	3.2	23.2	0.79
Rhubarb & Custard Doughnut	4	207	3.5	29.9	5.00
ASDA Extra Special Salted Caramel Donuts	2	211	3.7	33.1	1.50
Sainsbury's Strawberry Jam & Cream Doughnuts	2	184	3.8	23.4	1.30

COMMON FOOD   DONUTS

Suggested Brands	Size (pack)	Kcal	S.fat (g)	Carbs (g)	£
Tesco Cream & Strawberry Jam Doughnuts	2	184	3.8	23.4	1.40
ASDA Chocolate Indulgence Donuts	2	197	3.8	28.4	1.50
Raspberry & Rose Doughnut	4	209	4.0	32.1	5.00
Lemon Doughnut	4	206	4.5	28.9	5.00
ASDA Free From 6 Donuts	6	212	4.5	26.1	1.40
Waitrose Strawberry Jam & Cream Doughnuts	2	188	4.6	21.6	2.00
ASDA 4 Jam & Cream Donuts	4	195	4.7	22.6	1.00
ASDA Raspberry & White Chocolate Donuts	2	224	4.9	31.9	1.50
ASDA Baker's Selection Mini Strawberry Donuts	18	221	5.0	29.6	1.00
10 Jam & Cream Donuts	10	189	5.2	25.4	1.65
Country Style 6 Real Dairy Cream & Jam Doughnuts	6	200	5.2	24.4	1.00
Sainsbury's Doughnuts Glazed Ring	4	214	5.3	24.8	1.00
Chocolate Praline Doughnut	4	244	5.3	28.1	5.00

COMMON FOOD   DONUTS

Suggested Brands	Size (pack)	Kcal	S.fat (g)	Carbs (g)	£
Tesco Toffee Doughnut	2	190	5.5	20.4	1.40
ASDA Baker's Selection 18 Mini Ring Donuts	18	237	5.5	28.4	1.00
Sainsbury's Raspberry Ripple Stripe Doughnuts	4	220	5.7	29.2	1.50
Sainsbury's Doughnuts White Iced Ring	4	222	6.0	26.9	1.00
Tesco Strawberry Ring Doughnut	18	241	6.1	29.9	1.00
Sainsbury's Doughnuts Chocolate Iced Ring	4	224	6.2	27.5	1.00
Sainsbury's Chocolate Striped Doughnuts	4	244	6.3	27.3	1.50
ASDA Baker's Selection Sugar Ring Donuts	5	223	6.4	21.5	0.79
ASDA Iced Donuts	12	234	6.4	26.1	2.50
ASDA Baker's Selection Mini Chocolate Donuts	18	237	6.4	27.8	1.00
Tesco Chocolate Mini Ring Doughnuts	18	242	6.4	28.8	1.00
Cadbury Chocolate Donuts	3	260	6.5	27.1	1.50
Morrisons Fresh Cream Jam Doughnuts	2	209	7.0	20.3	1.65

COMMON FOOD   DONUTS

Suggested Brands	Size (pack)	Kcal	S.fat (g)	Carbs (g)	£
Chocolate Iced Ring Doughnut	4	245	7.3	26.9	1.20
Strawberry Iced Ring Doughnut	4	248	7.4	26.3	1.20
Daim Donuts	3	251	7.4	28.1	1.50
Tesco Millionaire Filled Doughnuts	3	253	7.4	28.3	1.65
Tesco White Iced Doughnuts	4	251	7.6	26.4	1.20
Tesco Ring Doughnuts	12	251	7.6	26.4	2.50
Oreo Donuts	3	263	7.7	27.1	1.50
Cadbury Caramel Donuts	3	243	7.8	29.0	1.50
Tesco Chocolate & Hazelnut Filled Doughnuts	3	276	8.1	27.9	1.65

VALUES SHOWN PER 58 GRAMS DONUT

Flour

Suggested Brands	Size (g)	Kcal	S.fat (g)	Carbs (g)	£
Stockwell And Co. Self Raising	1500	348	0.05	74.6	0.45
Stockwell And Co. Plain	1500	349	0.05	74.3	0.45
ASDA Smart Price Self Raising	1500	348	0.1	75	0.45
ASDA Smart Price White Plain	1500	349	0.1	74	0.45
Homepride Self Raising	1000	340	0.14	72	1.50
Homepride Plain	1000	341	0.19	70.8	1.50
McDougalls Self Raising	1100	330	0.2	67.9	1.00
Hovis Malted Brown Granary	1000	334	0.2	68.6	1.80
Sainsbury's Self Raising Flour, Basics	1500	335	0.2	69.9	0.60
Sainsbury's Self Raising	1500	335	0.2	69.9	0.80
Tesco Plain	1500	340	0.2	70.4	0.60
McDougalls Plain	1100	340	0.2	70.1	1.00
Sainsbury's Plain Flour, Basics	1500	342	0.2	71.7	0.60
Sainsbury's Plain	1500	342	0.2	71.7	0.80
Allinson Strong White Bread	1500	342	0.2	68.6	2.00
Tesco Very Strong Canadian Bread	1000	344	0.2	68.1	1.25
ASDA Free From Self Raising	1000	345	0.2	79	1.50
ASDA Free From Gluten Free Plain	1000	347	0.2	80	1.50

Suggested Brands	Size (g)	Kcal	S.fat (g)	Carbs (g)	£
FREEE by Doves Farm Gluten Free White Bread Flour	1000	351	0.2	79.8	1.68
McDougalls Supreme Sponge Premium Self Raising	1000	383	0.2	76.7	1.99
McDougalls 00 Grade Premium Plain	1000	399	0.2	84.7	1.79
Waitrose dark rye	1000	320	0.3	57.9	1.49
Doves Farm Organic Strong White	1500	335	0.3	67.4	2.00
Morrisons Self Raising	1500	338	0.3	69.3	0.80
Waitrose Duchy Organic stoneground plain wholemeal	1500	338	0.3	63.9	1.99
Doves Farm Organic White	1000	339	0.3	71.3	1.75
Sainsbury's Strong Brown	1500	340	0.3	61.8	1.00
Allinson Wholemeal Seed & Grain Bread	1000	340	0.3	58.3	1.50
Carrs Breadmaker Strong White	1500	340	0.3	68.7	1.50
Morrisons 00 Flour	500	344	0.3	70.7	0.65
Sainsbury's Strong White Unbleached Bread	1500	344	0.3	68.2	1.05
Sainsbury's Very Strong Canadian Bread Flour,	1000	346	0.3	67.3	1.10
Morrisons Strong White	1500	347	0.3	68.6	1.00
ASDA Strong White Bread	1500	348	0.3	70	0.69
Tesco Strong White	1500	348	0.3	69.9	1.00

COMMON FOOD   FLOUR

Suggested Brands	Size (g)	Kcal	S.fat (g)	Carbs (g)	£
FREEE by Doves Farm Self Raising White Flour Free From Gluten	1000	348	0.3	79.8	1.65
Waitrose Duchy Organic strong white bread	1500	349	0.3	69.5	1.89
ASDA Self Raising	1500	352	0.3	73	0.54
Tesco Self Raising	1500	352	0.3	73	0.60
Morrisons Organic Self Raising	1000	353	0.3	70.1	1.25
FREEE by Doves Farm Plain White Flour Free From Gluten	1000	353	0.3	79.9	1.65
Doves Farm Gluten Free Plain	1000	353	0.3	79.9	1.75
ASDA Plain	1500	357	0.3	74	0.54
ASDA Organic White Bread	1000	360	0.3	72	1.29
Waitrose Duchy Organic self raising white	1500	360	0.3	73.2	1.89
Tesco Organic Plain	1000	361	0.3	73	1.25
New - Morrisons Organic Plain	1000	361	0.3	73	1.25
Carrs Breadmaker Wholemeal	1500	316	0.4	58.9	1.50
Allinson Self-Raising Wholemeal	1000	326	0.4	60	1.94
Doves Farm Organic Spelt	1000	330	0.4	63.6	2.20
Morrisons Brown	1500	340	0.4	64.3	1.15
Morrisons Plain	1500	344	0.4	70.3	0.80
ASDA Organic Wholemeal Bread	1000	344	0.4	60	1.29

COMMON FOOD FLOUR

Suggested Brands	Size (g)	Kcal	S.fat (g)	Carbs (g)	£
Allinson Seed & Grain White	1000	344	0.4	66.7	1.50
Waitrose Canadian & very strong white bread	1500	348	0.4	67.4	1.79
ASDA Brown Bread	1500	351	0.4	64	0.79
Tesco Strong Brown Bread	1500	351	0.4	64.4	1.00
Allinson Very Strong Bread	1500	351	0.4	67	1.97
Waitrose Duchy Organic strong malted grain bread	1500	351	0.4	68.4	2.25
KTC Super Fine Gram	1000	352	0.4	55	1.40
Leckford Estate self raising white	1500	352	0.4	71.3	1.59
Waitrose spelt	1000	352	0.4	66.6	1.99
Waitrose Duchy Organic plain white	1500	363	0.4	73.5	1.89
Allinson Wholemeal Very Strong Bread	1500	333	0.5	59	1.97
Waitrose Canadian & strong stoneground wholemeal bread	1500	335	0.5	57	1.79
Waitrose Duchy Organic stoneground strong wholemeal bread	1500	337	0.5	59.4	1.99
ASDA Wholemeal Bread	1500	346	0.5	60	0.69
Leckford Estate plain white	1500	346	0.5	68.9	1.59
Allinson Plain Wholemeal	1000	350	0.5	65	1.94
FREEE by Doves Farm Rice Flour Free From Gluten	1000	354	0.5	75.2	1.65
Leckford Estate strong white bread	1500	354	0.5	69.7	1.79

Suggested Brands	Size (g)	Kcal	S.fat (g)	Carbs (g)	£
Waitrose Duchy Organic self raising brown	1500	359	0.5	69.8	1.99
Waitrose LoveLife Calorie Controlled crunchy mixed seed bread	1500	373	0.5	69	1.99
Tesco Strong Stone Ground 100% Wholemeal Bread	1500	333	0.6	59.4	1.10
essential Waitrose strong wholemeal bread	1500	333	0.6	59.3	1.19
Doves Farm Wholemeal Buckwheat	1000	335	0.6	65.4	3.00
Sharpham Park spelt & rye	1000	340	0.6	62.5	2.75
Sharpham Park organic spelt stoneground	1000	349	0.6	60	3.59
Waitrose LoveLife Calorie Controlled seeded wholemeal bread	1500	353	0.6	55.6	1.99
Suryaa Wheat	1000	354	0.6	75.2	1.69
Sharpham Park Organic spelt flour artisan	1000	344	0.78	64	3.49
Sharpham Park organic spelt flour wholegrain	1000	340	0.9	60	3.49
essential Waitrose self-raising white wheat	1500	350	0.9	72.3	0.92
essential Waitrose strong white bread wheat	1500	361	0.9	71.7	1.15
Sainsbury's Wholegrain Seeded Flour, Taste the Difference	1000	365	0.9	56.9	1.10

Common Food   Flour

Suggested Brands	Size (g)	Kcal	S.fat (g)	Carbs (g)	£
essential Waitrose strong brown bread	1500	366	0.9	72.3	1.09
Waitrose LoveLife Calorie Controlled seeded & malted bread	1500	397	0.9	67.5	1.99
essential Waitrose plain white	1500	352	1.4	71.2	0.92
Biona Organic Coconut	500	339	8.0	46	3.98
The Groovy Food Company Organic Coconut Flour	500	352	11	16	3.76
Groovy Food Organic Coconut	500	352	11	16	3.85

Values Shown Is Per 100 Grams

Your Favourite Food Not Included?
Let Us Know

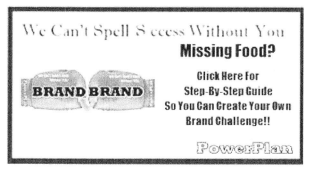

WWW.WECANTSPELLSUCCESSWITHOUTYOU.COM

Ice Cream

Suggested Brands	Size (g)	Kcal	S.fat (g)	Carbs (g)	£
Sainsbury's Sorbet Mango	500	27.9	0.1	6.4	2.20
Halo Top Sea Salt Caramel	473	23.1	0.3	4.8	3.50
Breyers Delights Salted Caramel Cake Lower Calorie	500	23.1	0.3	3.4	5.00
Morrisons Low Calorie High Protein Peanut Butter	480	24.1	0.3	3.9	2.50
ASDA Smart Price Vanilla Soft Scoop	2000	19.4	0.4	2.7	0.92
Halo Top Peanut Butter Cup	473	23.1	0.4	4.1	3.50
Halo Top Red Velvet	472	25.8	0.4	4.8	3.50
Morrisons Low Calorie High Protein Choc Chip Cookie Dough	480	24.5	0.5	3.1	2.50
Halo Top Chocolate Chip Cookie Dough	473	25.8	0.5	4.8	3.50
Morrisons Vanilla	2000	23.1	0.7	3.3	1.65
Carte D'or Vanilla Light	1000	24.5	0.7	3.7	3.50
Morrisons Neapolitan	2000	23.8	0.8	3.4	1.65
Morrisons Raspberry Ripple	2000	26.2	0.8	4.0	1.65
Tesco Neapolitan	1000	39.4	0.8	6.3	1.00
Walls Soft Scoop Vanilla	1800	27.9	0.9	3.4	2.20
Carte D'or Strawberry	1000	30.9	0.9	5.1	3.50
Carte D'or Rum & Raisin	1000	34.0	0.9	4.4	3.50
Carte D'or Salted Caramel	1000	34.0	1.0	5.1	3.50
Tesco Soft Scoop Vanilla	2000	51.7	1.1	8.2	1.50

COMMON FOOD   ICE CREAM

Suggested Brands	Size (g)	Kcal	S.fat (g)	Carbs (g)	£
Tesco Soft Scoop Neapolitan	2000	51.7	1.1	8.3	1.50
ASDA Really Creamy Vanilla	900	31.3	1.2	4.1	1.68
Morrisons Double Chocolate	900	36.7	1.2	5.3	2.00
Essential Waitrose vanilla & raspberry ripple	1000	37.1	1.2	5.5	1.65
Carte D'or Mint Chocolate	1000	37.1	1.2	4.8	3.50
Morrisons Toffee & Vanilla Ice	900	37.7	1.2	5.6	2.00
Morrisons Strawberry & Cream	900	35.4	1.3	4.8	2.00
essential Waitrose vanilla soft	1000	36.7	1.3	5.0	1.30
essential Waitrose vanilla soft ice cream	2000	36.7	1.3	5.0	2.00
ASDA Triple Chocolate	900	38.1	1.3	5.1	1.68
ASDA Galactic	900	38.8	1.3	5.8	2.00
Sainsbury's Vanilla Soft Scoop	2000	41.8	1.3	6.3	1.80
Sainsbury's Neapolitan Soft Scoop	2000	42.5	1.3	6.2	1.80
Tesco White Chocolate & Raspberry	900	46.9	1.3	6.8	2.00
Tesco Triple Chocolate	900	51.9	1.3	7.5	2.00
Morrisons Vanilla Ice Cream	900	33.0	1.4	4.3	2.00
ASDA Unicorn	900	39.8	1.4	6.1	2.00
Morrisons Salted Caramel	900	40.1	1.4	5.8	2.00

Suggested Brands	Size (g)	Kcal	S.fat (g)	Carbs (g)	£
ASDA Really Creamy Mint Choc Chip	900	44.2	1.4	6.1	1.68
Sainsbury's Chocolate Soft Scoop	2000	44.5	1.4	6.5	1.80
Ms Molly's Vanilla	2000	68.7	1.4	10.9	0.99
Carte D'or Indulgent Chocolate	1000	39.1	1.5	4.4	3.50
Morrisons Mint Chocolate Chip	900	39.8	1.5	5.5	2.00
Morrisons Caramel Latte	900	40.8	1.5	6.0	2.00
Iceland Soft Scoop Vanilla	2000	43.5	1.5	6.2	1.50
Iceland Neapolitan Soft Scoop	2000	44.9	1.5	6.4	1.50
Iceland Made in Italy Caramel Swirl	900	51.7	1.5	8.4	1.75
Tesco Caramel Vanilla	900	57.8	1.5	8.9	2.00
Sainsbury's Raspberry Ripple Soft Scoop	2000	43.5	1.6	6.1	1.80
Maltesers	500	43.5	1.7	5.8	3.00
ASDA Really Creamy Caramel Fudge	900	45.2	1.7	6.1	1.68
Mackies Traditional Luxury Dairy	1000	53.0	1.8	6.0	3.00
Tesco Cornish	2000	51.9	1.9	5.4	3.00
Tesco Vanilla Ice Cream	900	51.9	2.0	5.5	2.00
ASDA Vanilla Soft Scoop	2000	56.8	2.0	8.0	1.35
ASDA Neapolitan Soft Scoop	2000	57.5	2.0	8.1	1.55
Oreo Ice Cream	480	61.2	2.2	7.8	2.25
Tesco Mint Chocolate	900	61.2	2.3	7.6	2.00
Carte D'Or Classic Vanilla	1000	67.0	2.3	10.2	3.50

COMMON FOOD   ICE CREAM

Suggested Brands	Size (g)	Kcal	S.fat (g)	Carbs (g)	£
Cadbury Flake	480	69.7	2.3	7.8	2.50
Kelly's Cornish Honeycomb Crunch	950	79.9	2.4	10.3	2.50
Cadbury Double Decker	480	57.5	2.6	6.4	3.00
Ben & Jerry's Chocolate Fudge Brownie	500	83.3	2.7	9.9	3.00
Ben & Jerry's Phish Food	500	91.8	2.7	12.2	3.00
Ben & Jerry's Cookie Dough	500	91.8	3.1	10.2	3.00
Kelly's Cornish Clotted Cream	1000	77.5	3.3	6.8	2.50
Haagen-Dazs Vanilla	460	85.3	3.5	6.8	2.50
Haagen-Dazs Salted Caramel	460	95.9	3.7	9.5	2.50
Haagen-Dazs Belgian Chocolate	460	106.8	4.3	8.9	2.50
Magnum Vegan Classic	270	112.2	4.8	11.6	3.50

VALUES SHOWN PER 34 GRAM SCOOP

Milk

Suggested Brands	Size (g)	Kcal	S.fat (g)	Carbs (g)	£
Morrisons Savers Long Life Skimmed Milk	1 Litre	33	0	4.5	0.52
Sainsbury's Skimmed Long Life Milk	1 Litre	33	0	4.5	0.80
Morrisons British Skimmed Milk	4 Pints	35	0.05	4.9	1.09
essential Waitrose skimmed milk 0.1% fat 4 pints	4 Pints	35	0.05	5	1.15
ASDA Skimmed Milk	4 Pints	37	0.05	5	1.09
Sainsbury's British Skimmed Milk	4 Pints	37	0.05	5	1.10
Viva Long Life UHT Skimmed Milk	1 Litre	34	0.06	4.9	0.65
ASDA Longlife Skimmed Milk	1 Litre	35	0.1	4.9	0.69
Iceland Fresh Pasteurised Skimmed Milk	4 Pints	35	0.1	5	1.80
ASDA Smart Price Longlife Skimmed Milk	1 Litre	37	0.1	4.9	0.52
Tesco Skimmed Longlife Milk	1 Litre	37	0.1	5.0	0.79
Arla Bob Skimmed Milk	2 Litre	41	0.1	4.9	1.55
Arla Lactofree Fresh Skimmed Milk	1 Litre	31	0.3	2.8	1.00

COMMON FOOD MILK

Suggested Brands	Size (g)	Kcal	S.fat (g)	Carbs (g)	£
Alpro Dairy Free Soya Original Longlife Milk Alternative	1 Litre	44	0.3	3	1.40
Morrisons British 1% Fat Milk	4 Pints	41	0.6	4.6	1.09
ASDA 1% Fat Milk	4 Pints	43	0.6	5	1.09
Sainsbury's British 1% Fat Milk	4 Pints	43	0.6	5	1.10
ASDA Lactose Free Semi Skimmed Milk Alternative	1 Litre	45	0.9	4.6	1.20
Arla Lactofree Fresh Semi Skimmed Milk	1 Litre	39	1.0	2.7	1.00
Moo Long Life Organic Milk, Semi Skimmed	1 Litre	46	1	4.6	0.80
Sainsbury's Semi Skimmed Long Life Milk	1 Litre	47	1	4.6	0.80
A2 Fresh Semi Skimmed Milk	1 Litre	48	1	4.7	1.40
Cravendale Semi Skimmed Milk	1 Litre	49	1.0	4.8	1.00
Morrisons British Semi Skimmed Milk	4 Pints	49	1	4.8	1.09
Morrisons For Farmers British Semi Skimmed Milk	4 Pints	49	1	4.8	1.32
Cravendale Purefilter Semi Skimmed Milk	2 Litre	49	1	4.8	1.50
Cravendale Semi Skimmed Milk	2 litre	49	1	4.8	1.75
M Organic British Semi Skimmed Milk	4 Pints	49	1	4.8	1.80

Suggested Brands	Size (g)	Kcal	S.fat (g)	Carbs (g)	£
Iceland Pasteurised Homogenised Semi Skimmed Milk	4 Pints	49	1	5	1.80
St Helen's Farm Semi Skimmed Goats Milk	1 Litre	44	1.1	4.3	1.75
Viva Long Life UHT Semi-Skimmed Milk	1 Litre	47	1.1	4.8	0.65
Waitrose Filtered Semi Skimmed Milk	2 Litre	47	1.1	4.6	0.90
Arla Organic Free Range Semi Skimmed Milk	2 Litre	47	1.1	4.8	1.75
Arla Semi-Skimmed Organic Fre range Milk	2 litre	47	1.1	4.8	1.75
Asda Arla Farmers Semi Skimmed Milk	4 Pints	48	1.1	4.7	1.34
Sainsbury's British Semi Skimmed Milk, SO Organic	4 Pints	48	1.1	4.6	1.80
ASDA Longlife Semi Skimmed Milk	1 Litre	50	1.1	4.8	0.69
Tesco Semi Skimmed Longlife Milk	1 Litre	50	1.1	4.8	0.79
Tesco Organic Semi-Skimmed Milk	2 Pints	50	1.1	4.8	0.89
ASDA Semi Skimmed Milk	4 Pints	50	1.1	4.8	1.09
Sainsbury's British Semi Skimmed Milk	4 Pints	50	1.1	4.8	1.10
Waitrose Duchy Organic semi-skimmed milk un-homogenised	1 Litre	50	1.1	4.8	1.15

Suggested Brands	Size (g)	Kcal	S.fat (g)	Carbs (g)	£
ASDA Organic Semi Skimmed Milk	4 Pints	50	1.1	4.8	1.50
Camelicious Long Life Whole Camel Milk (DB type 1)	235ml	221	1.7	4.4	3.05
Arla Organic Kefir Natural Cultured Milk Drink	1 Litre	59	1.9	3.9	2.00
A2 Milk Whole	1 Litre	67	2.2	4.9	1.40
Arla Lactofree Fresh Whole Milk	1 Litre	56	2.3	2.6	1.00
Sainsbury's Whole Long Life Milk	1 Litre	64	2.3	4.6	1.00
Asda Arla Farmers Whole Milk	4 Pints	64	2.3	4.6	1.34
Iceland British Fresh Pasteurised Whole Milk	4 Pints	64	2.3	4.7	1.80
ASDA Longlife Whole Milk	1 Litre	65	2.3	4.7	0.69
Viva Whole Milk	1 Litre	65	2.3	4.7	0.70
Cravendale Whole Milk	1 Litre	65	2.3	4.7	1.00
Morrisons British Whole Milk	4 Pints	65	2.3	4.7	1.09
Cravendale Whole Milk	2 litre	65	2.3	4.7	1.75
St Helen's Farm Whole Goats Milk	1 Litre	61	2.4	4.3	1.75
Waitrose Filtered Whole Milk	2 Litre	65	2.4	4.8	0.90

COMMON FOOD   MILK

Suggested Brands	Size (g)	Kcal	S.fat (g)	Carbs (g)	£
Tesco Whole Longlife Milk	1 Litre	66	2.4	4.7	0.79
ASDA Whole Milk	4 Pints	66	2.4	4.7	1.09
Tesco Whole Milk	4 Pints	66	2.4	4.7	1.09
Sainsbury's British Whole Milk	4 Pints	66	2.4	4.7	1.10
ASDA Organic Whole Milk	4 Pints	69	2.4	4.7	1.50
Arla Big Milk Added Vitamins Whole Milk	2 Litre	68	2.6	4.7	1.75
Arla Organic Free Range Whole Milk	2 Litre	68	2.6	4.7	1.75
M Organic British Whole Milk	4 Pints	68	2.6	4.7	1.80
Morrisons The Best Unhomogenised Jersey Milk	1 Litre	79	3.2	4.6	1.15
Graham's Gold Jersey Milk	1 Litre	81	3.4	4.7	1.10
Arla B.O.B Fat Free Skimmed Milk	2 litre	41	9.1	4.9	1.25

VALUES SHOWN PER 100 ML

Mousse

Suggested Brands	Size (g)	Kcal	S.fat (g)	Carbs (g)	£
Sainsbury's Mousse Lighter Chocolate x 6	375	71.9	0.9	10.5	1.00
ASDA Light Chocolate x 6	360	65.4	1.0	9.6	1.00
Tesco Healthy Living Chocolate x 6	360	69.6	1.0	10.7	1.00
Nestle Aero Chocolate x 4	236	93.8	1.8	13.6	1.00
Ski Lemon with Meringue Sauce x 6	360	76.8	1.9	10.7	1.00
Ski Strawberry x 6	360	72.6	2.0	9.2	1.00
Rolo x 4	200	79.0	2.1	10.8	1.00
ASDA Smart Price Chocolate x 6	360	67.8	2.2	10.8	0.45
Ms Molly's Chocolate x 4	240	79.8	2.3	10.9	1.00
Milkybar Mousses x 4	210	81.4	2.3	9.9	1.00
Aero Mint Chocolate x 4	192	82.1	2.5	10.3	1.00
Cadbury Bubbles of Joy Milk Chocolate x 4	180	90.0	2.6	11.5	1.00
essential Waitrose chocolate x 6	375	106.9	2.8	13.4	1.00
Cadbury Layers of Joy Jaffantastic Chocolate x 2	180	186.3	3.2	31.9	0.80
Iceland 6 Chocolate	330	101.8	3.3	12.8	1.20
Bonne Maman Strawberry x 2	140	120.4	3.3	16.1	1.00
Tesco Chocolate x 6	360	104.4	3.4	13.4	0.49
ASDA Chocolate Mousses x 6	360	104.4	3.4	13.2	1.00
Morrisons Chocolate x 6	360	104.4	3.4	13.4	1.40
Sainsbury's Chocolate x 6	360	111.0	3.6	14.0	1.50

COMMON FOOD   MOUSSE

Suggested Brands	Size (g)	Kcal	S.fat (g)	Carbs (g)	£
Somerset Valley Strawberry x 6	330	86.9	3.9	9.3	1.00
ASDA Lemon x 6	360	107.4	4.1	13.8	1.40
Tesco Mousse x 6	360	107.4	4.1	13.7	1.50
Morrisons Lemon x 6	360	107.4	4.1	13.7	1.50
Tesco Strawberry x 6	360	93.6	4.3	10.1	1.00
ASDA Strawberry Mousses x 6	360	93.6	4.3	10.2	1.00
Aero Creations Chocolate x 4	228	130.0	5.2	11.7	1.00
Nestle After Eight x 4	228	126.0	5.5	10.3	1.00
Waitrose Lemon x 1	100	166.0	6.5	13.8	1.00
Waitrose cappuccino x 1	100	200.0	6.6	21.6	1.50
Muller Pud Belgian Chocolate x 1	200	354.0	7.8	49.6	1.40
Muller Pud Belgian Chocolate and Orange x 1	200	354.0	7.8	49.6	1.50
Tesco Finest Cherry & Kirsch x 1	100	195.0	7.9	19.6	1.00
GU Dark Chocolate and Salted Caramel x 1	70	247.1	8.3	26.5	1.75
GU Intense Chocolate x 1	70	225.4	8.8	20.8	1.75
ASDA Red Berry x 2	200	217.0	9.2	18.0	1.00
Muller Püd Mousse Belgian Chocolate and White Chocolate x 1	200	358.0	9.2	49.2	1.50
Bonne Maman Chocolate x 2	140	206.5	9.9	13.2	0.80
Waitrose Chocolate x 1	100	261.0	9.9	23.2	0.65
ASDA Toffee x 2	200	235.0	10.0	21.0	0.80

COMMON FOOD MOUSSE

Suggested Brands	Size (g)	Kcal	S.fat (g)	Carbs (g)	£
Tesco Finest Mango & Passion Fruit x 1	100	231.0	10.3	18.4	0.80
Morrisons The Best Snowdonia Fudge x 1	100	252.0	10.4	25.3	0.80
Sainsbury's Salted Caramel Mousse, Taste the Difference x 1	100	246.0	10.8	19.2	0.80
Finest Butter Scotch x 1	100	270.0	11.1	26.0	0.80
Sainsbury's Mousse Colombian Coffee, Taste the Difference x 1	100	271.0	11.5	23.8	0.80
Tesco Finest Belgian Chocolate x 1	100	285.0	11.6	23.9	0.80
Sainsbury's Mousse Chocolate, Taste the Difference x 1	100	313.0	12.4	29.8	0.80
Morrisons The Best Belgian Chocolate x 1	100	307.0	12.8	25.5	0.65

VALUES SHOWN PER POT

Noodles

(Instant and Super, Excluding Pot Snacks)

Suggested Brands	Size (g)	Kcal	S.fat (g)	Carbs (g)	£
Amoy Straight to Wok Udon Thick Noodles	150	425	0.0	86.1	0.90
Amoy Straight To Wok Ribbon Rice Noodles Gluten Free	150	432	0.0	104.5	0.90
Blue Dragon Medium Egg Noodles Nests (boiled)	300	362	0.5	71	1.50
Sharwood's Medium Egg Noodles (boiled)	340	367	0.5	71.2	3.75
Amoy straight to wok noodles thread	150	429	1.0	75.4	0.90
Amoy straight to wok medium noodles	150	506	1.0	91.5	0.90
Amoy Straight to Wok Singapore Noodles	150	459	1.3	72.4	0.90
Tesco Instant Noodles Chow Mein Flavoured	85	446	4.7	60.3	0.30
ASDA Egg Noodles (boiled)	250	251	5.0	36.9	0.59
Mama Hot & Spicy Flavour Oriental Style Instant Noodles	90	251	5.0	36.9	0.70
Kimchi Oriental Style Instant Noodle	90	251	5.0	36.9	0.70
Mama Oriental Style Instant Noodles Shrimp Creamy Tom Yum Flavour	90	251	5.0	63.7	0.70
Mama Instant Noodles Chicken Flavour	70	271	5.0	39.5	1.00

Koka Instant Noodles Chicken Flavour	85	271	5.4	34.8	0.45
Koka Instant Noodles Curry Flavour	85	271	5.4	35.2	0.45
Koka Instant Noodles Vegetable Flavour	85	271	5.4	35.2	0.45
MAGGI 3 Minute Instant Chicken Flavour Noodle	59	273	5.4	30	0.25
Tesco Chicken Flavour Instant Noodles	85	513	5.4	73.7	0.30
Mama Instant Noodles Shrimp Tom Yum Flavour	70	285	5.7	39.5	1.00
Indo Mie Instant Special Chicken Flavour Noodles	75	350	6	48.1	0.45
ASDA Smart Price Chicken Instant Noodles	65	372	7.0	50.3	0.20
Indo Mie Instant Noodles Pepper Chicken Flavor	70	400	7	53	0.40
Indo Mie Instant Noodles Chicken Curry Flavour	80	455	7.2	65.4	0.45
ASDA Instant Curry Noodles	85	446	8.0	57.0	0.22
ASDA Instant Curry Noodles	85	446	8.0	57.0	0.22
Indo Mie Instant Special Chicken Flavour Noodles	75	466	8	64.1	0.40
Indo Mie Instant Noodles Mi Goreng Hot & Spicy	80	480	8.4	65.3	0.40
ASDA Instant Chicken Noodles	85	472	8.7	67.0	0.22
ASDA Instant Chicken Noodles	85	472	8.7	67.0	0.22

Indo Mie Instant Noodles Soup Vegetable Flavour with Lime	75	476	8.9	61.4	0.45
Mama Oriental Style Instant Noodles Green Curry Flavour	90	454	9	64	0.70
Morrisons Instant Noodles BBQ Beef	85	466	9.4	59.3	0.28
MAGGI 3 Minute Instant BBQ Beef Flavour Noodle	59	457	9.9	61.4	0.25
Morrisons Mild Curry Instant Noodles	85	459	10.1	56.6	0.28
Morrisons Bacon Flavour Instant Noodles	85	489	10.1	63.7	0.28
Batchelors Super Noodles Bacon Flavour	90	506	10.4	65.0	0.50
Batchelors Super Noodles Chicken Flavour	90	506	10.4	65.3	0.50
Batchelors Super Noodles BBQ Beef Flavour	90	506	10.4	65.3	0.50
Batchelors Super Noodles Southern Fried Chicken Flavour	90	509	10.4	65.3	0.50
Batchelors Super Noodles Chicken & Mushroom Flavour	90	513	10.4	65.7	0.50
Batchelors Super Noodles Chow Mein Flavour	90	513	10.4	66.3	0.50
Batchelors Super Noodles Curry Flavour	90	519	10.4	67.3	0.50
Wai Wai Instant Noodles Casserole Beef Flavour	60	494	11	61	0.45

COMMON FOOD   NOODLES

Wai Wai Oriental Style Instant Noodles	60	501	11	62	0.45
Wai Wai Instant Noodles Chicken Flavour	60	504	11	61	0.45
Wai Wai Instant Noodles Chicken Flavour	60	504	11	61	0.45
Morrisons Instant Noodles Chicken	85	526	11.4	64.7	0.28
Sainsbury's Instant Noodles, Chicken, Basics	90	586	13.1	71.7	0.25
Sainsbury's Instant Noodles, Chicken	85	586	13.1	71.7	0.45
Sainsbury's Instant Noodles, BBQ	85	590	13.1	71.7	0.45
Sainsbury's Instant Noodles, Curry	85	590	13.1	72.0	0.45
Indo Mie Mi Goreng Halal Instant Fried Noodles	80	754	19.8	96.5	0.40
Indo Mie Mi Goreng Halal Instant Fried Noodles	80	383	49	10.1	0.40

VALUES SHOWN PER PACKET EATEN WHEN WATER ADDED TO 335 GRAMS

Pasta

Suggested Brands	Size (g)	Kcal	S.fat (g)	Carbs (g)	£
ASDA Smart Price Pasta Shapes	500	88.2	0.0	18.0	0.29
ASDA Farfalle	500	93.6	0.0	18.6	0.65
M Organic Fusilli	500	76.2	0.1	15.6	1.00
ASDA Tricolore Fusilli	500	85.8	0.1	17.4	0.65
ASDA 50 50 Fusilli	500	85.8	0.1	16.2	0.75
ASDA Wholewheat Penne	500	88.8	0.1	16.8	0.53
ASDA Penne	500	93.0	0.1	18.6	0.53
ASDA Orzo	500	93.0	0.1	18.6	0.65
ASDA Tagliatelle	500	93.0	0.1	18.6	0.75
Morrisons Fusilli	500	93.6	0.1	18.7	0.61
Morrisons Conchiglie	500	93.6	0.1	18.7	0.61
Sainsbury's Tagliatelle	500	96.6	0.1	19.7	0.70
Sainsbury's Pasta Shapes, Basics	500	97.2	0.1	19.6	0.30
Seeds of Change organic spinach trottole pasta	500	97.2	0.1	20.1	2.30
Seeds Of Change Organic Trottole	500	97.2	0.1	20.1	2.40
Seeds of Change organic tortiglioni semi wholewheat pasta	500	99.0	0.1	20.1	2.30
Seeds of Change organic penne pasta	500	99.6	0.1	20.1	2.30
Tesco Whole Wheat Fusilli	500	100.8	0.1	19.7	0.50
Tesco Whole Wheat Penne	500	100.8	0.1	19.7	0.50
Tesco Finest Orzo Pasta	500	102.0	0.1	20.3	1.70

Suggested Brands	Size (g)	Kcal	S.fat (g)	Carbs (g)	£
Morrisons Free From Fusilli	500	103.2	0.1	23.2	1.20
Hearty Food Co. Penne Pasta	500	104.4	0.1	21.7	0.29
Tesco Fusilli	500	105.0	0.1	21.4	0.50
Tesco Conchiglie shells	500	105.0	0.1	21.4	0.50
Tesco Dischi Volanti	500	105.0	0.1	21.4	0.50
Tesco Spirali Pasta	500	105.6	0.1	21.4	0.50
Tesco Rigatoni	500	105.6	0.1	21.4	0.50
Tesco Tagliatelle	500	105.6	0.1	21.4	0.50
Tesco Macaroni	500	105.6	0.1	21.4	0.50
Morrisons The Best Trotolle	500	108.6	0.1	21.5	1.70
Morrisons The Best Fusilli Gigante	500	108.6	0.1	21.5	1.70
Morrisons The Best Conchiglioni	500	108.6	0.1	21.5	1.70
De Cecco Penne Rigate	500	117.6	0.1	23.4	1.55
De Cecco pasta penne rigate	500	117.6	0.1	23.4	1.55
Tesco Free From Fusilli	500	118.2	0.1	26.2	1.00
Tesco Free From Penne	500	118.2	0.1	26.2	1.00
De Cecco pasta chifferi rigati	500	118.2	0.1	24.4	1.55
Napolina Penne	500	118.8	0.1	24.0	1.50
Napolina Fusilli	500	121.8	0.1	24.0	1.00
Waitrose 1 paccheri rigati pasta tubes	500	123.0	0.1	24.4	1.70
Morrisons Wholewheat Fusiili	500	85.8	0.2	16.2	0.61

Suggested Brands	Size (g)	Kcal	S.fat (g)	Carbs (g)	£
Sainsbury's Fresh Egg Fusilli	500	90.6	0.2	16.1	1.70
Sainsbury's Fresh Egg Penne	500	90.6	0.2	16.1	1.70
essential Waitrose fresh pasta fusilli	500	96.6	0.2	17.8	1.70
essential Waitrose fresh pasta penne	500	96.6	0.2	17.8	1.70
essential Waitrose fresh pasta tagliatelle	500	96.6	0.2	17.8	1.70
Sainsbury's Deliciously Free From Fusilli	500	102.0	0.2	21.6	1.25
Filiz Pasta Pipe Rigate	500	119.4	0.2	24.4	0.69
Barilla Mezze Penne Tricolore	500	119.4	0.2	23.6	0.85
Barilla Fusilli Pasta	500	119.4	0.2	23.8	0.85
Sainsbury's Fresh Egg Tagliatelle	500	99.0	0.3	18.3	1.30
Waitrose wholewheat fresh pasta tagliatelle	500	87.0	0.4	13.1	1.70
Sainsbury's Wholewheat Penne	500	94.2	0.5	18.1	0.55
Sainsbury's Wholewheat Fusilli, SO Organic	500	94.2	0.5	18.1	1.00
Sainsbury's Farfalle	500	96.0	0.5	19.5	0.55
Sainsbury's Conchiglie (Shells)	500	96.0	0.5	19.5	0.55
Sainsbury's Spirali	500	96.0	0.5	19.5	0.55
Sainsbury's Macaroni	500	96.0	0.5	19.5	0.55
Sainsbury's Fusilli	500	96.0	0.5	19.5	0.55

COMMON FOOD   PASTA

Suggested Brands	Size (g)	Kcal	S.fat (g)	Carbs (g)	£
Sainsbury's Rigatoni (tubes),	500	96.0	0.5	19.5	0.55
Sainsbury's Penne Rigate	500	96.0	0.5	19.5	0.55
Sainsbury's Orzo	500	96.0	0.5	19.5	0.55
Sainsbury's Fusilli Tricolori	500	96.0	0.5	19.5	0.70

VALUES SHOWN PER 60 GRAMS UNCOOKED

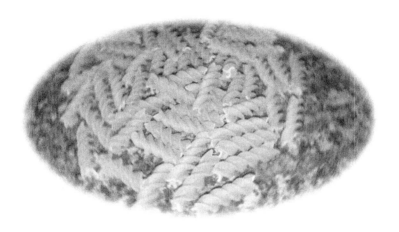

Pizza (Whole)

Suggested Brands	Size (g)	Kcal	S.fat (g)	Carbs (g)	£
ASDA Cheese & Ham Pizza	114	303.2	2.3	43.3	0.61
No Cheese Italian Garden	382	744.9	3.1	110.8	2.00
ASDA Cheese & Tomato Pizza	110	294.8	3.6	40.7	0.61
No Cheese Houmous	284	701.5	4.5	68.2	2.00
Sainsbury's Cheese & Tomato Pizza, Basics 7"	119	365.3	5.1	48.7	0.75
ASDA Smart Price Cheese & Tomato	268	627.1	5.4	93.8	0.60
Morrisons Sweet Chilli Chicken Extra Thin	362	988.3	5.8	119.8	1.50
Morrisons BBQ Chicken Sourdough	395	837.4	6.3	112.2	1.50
Pizza Express La Reine	290	611.9	6.7	80.3	5.00
Iceland Vegetable Thin	329	756.7	7.2	98.4	1.00
Tesco Stonebaked Thin Sweet Chilli Chicken	330	739.2	7.3	99.7	1.50
Morrisons 2 Pepperoni Pizza Baguettes	225	504.0	7.7	62.8	1.00
Pizza Express Vegan Giardiniera	272	549.4	7.9	82.4	5.00
Chicago Town 3 Cheese & Tomato Pizza Toasties	225	643.5	8.1	83.3	1.65
Iceland Southern Spiced Chicken Thin	336	840.0	8.1	102.5	1.00
Iceland Ham & Mushroom Deep Pan	413	900.3	8.3	133.0	1.00

Suggested Brands	Size (g)	Kcal	S.fat (g)	Carbs (g)	£
Iceland Chicken Fajita Thin	335	807.4	8.4	99.8	1.00
Iceland Barbecue Chicken Thin	334	855.0	8.4	111.9	1.00
Morrisons Ham & Pineapple Thin & Crispy	315	762.3	8.5	109.9	2.00
Morrisons Spicy Chicken Thin & Crispy	320	732.8	8.6	98.6	2.00
Morrisons Cheese & Ham Thin	345	821.1	8.6	105.6	1.00
Morrisons The Best Chargrilled Vegetables	510	1101.6	8.7	147.4	4.00
Tesco Stonebaked Thin Bbq Meat Feast	340	856.8	8.8	116.6	1.50
ASDA Cheese & Tomato (Margherita) Thin & Crispy Pizza	330	831.6	8.9	108.9	0.90
Whole Creations Butternut Squash, Red Pepper & Caramelised Onion Sheesy	300	585.0	9.0	89.4	3.75
Morrisons Mediterranean Veg Extra Thin	375	821.3	9.0	85.9	1.50
Morrisons Mozzarella & Pesto Sourdough	353	900.2	9.2	110.1	1.50
Iceland Ham & Pineapple Thin	345	824.6	9.3	105.9	1.00
Chicago Town 2 Deep Dish Chicken Club	320	835.2	9.3	102.4	2.00
Sainsbury's Deep Pan BBQ Chicken	422	991.7	9.3	148.5	1.30

Suggested Brands	Size (g)	Kcal	S.fat (g)	Carbs (g)	£
ASDA Sweet Chilli Chicken Extra Thin & Crisp	375	810.0	9.4	90.0	1.20
Morrisons Thin Cheese	318	826.8	9.5	121.5	1.00
Hearty Food Thin Cheese And Tomato	314	788.1	9.7	111.5	0.67
Sainsbury's Stonebaked Chicken & Pesto Pizza 10"	315	746.6	9.8	80.3	2.00
Iceland Stonebaked Mediterranean Vegetable	408	758.9	9.8	110.6	1.59
ASDA Fajita Chicken Stonebaked 10"	330	689.7	9.9	79.2	1.87
Sainsbury's Thin & Crispy Hawaiian	413	883.8	9.9	121.4	1.40
Waitrose 1 wood-fired buffalo mozzarella & sun soaked tomato	295	764.1	10.0	97.1	3.89
Iceland Stonebaked BBQ Chicken & Bacon	345	769.4	10.0	103.8	1.59
Iceland Stonebaked Sweet Chilli Chicken	415	809.3	10.0	118.3	1.59
Waitrose Vegan Stonebaked Margherita	385	843.2	10.0	132.4	4.99
Sainsbury's Stonebaked Spinach & Ricotta Pizza 10'	320	726.4	10.2	91.2	3.00
Waitrose 1 wood-fired roasted vegetable & pesto	335	794.0	10.4	100.2	3.89
ASDA Cheese & Tomato 10"	257	696.5	10.5	87.4	1.11

Suggested Brands	Size (g)	Kcal	S.fat (g)	Carbs (g)	£
Tesco Stonebaked Ham And Pineapple	375	821.3	10.5	99.8	1.50
ASDA Mediterranean Vegetable Extra Thin & Crispy	375	952.5	10.5	21.4	1.20
Sainsbury's Vegetable	406	877.0	10.6	114.5	1.40
Iceland Double Cheeseburger Deep Pan	380	1003.2	10.6	138.7	1.00
Dr. Oetker Yes It's Pizza Spinach Based Broccoli & Mushroom	335	696.8	10.7	73.7	3.00
Hearty Food Thin Pepperoni	314	813.3	10.7	103.0	0.67
Waitrose hand stretched pepper & ricotta	430	1053.5	10.8	147.5	4.50
Goodfella's Romano Chicken, Roquito Pepper & Red Onion with a Garlic Oil Drizzle	389	918.0	10.9	101.1	2.50
Sainsbury's Stonebaked Ham & Pineapple Pizza 10"	305	719.8	11.0	87.2	2.00
Dr. Oetker Ristorante Thin & Crispy Pollo	355	791.7	11.0	92.3	2.50
Goodfella's Ham & Pineapple Thin	365	843.2	11.0	105.9	2.00
Iceland Chicken & Sweetcorn Pizza Deep Pan	411	953.5	11.1	125.8	1.00
Morrisons Savers Cheese & Tomato	220	567.6	11.2	68.2	0.95

Suggested Brands	Size (g)	Kcal	S.fat (g)	Carbs (g)	£
Sainsbury's Spicy Chicken	404	909.0	11.3	117.6	1.40
Iceland Cheese & Ham Thin	327	856.7	11.4	100.1	1.00
Sainsbury's Stonebaked Hot & Spicy Pizza 10"	320	723.2	11.5	81.0	3.00
ASDA Stonebaked BBQ Chicken	395	896.7	11.5	114.6	1.20
Waitrose hand stretched chicken & chorizo	395	1050.7	11.5	126.4	4.50
ASDA BBQ Chicken Deep Pan Pizza	423	968.7	11.8	135.4	0.90
The White Rabbit Pizza Co. Smokin' Vegan	340	741.2	11.9	106.4	5.00
Sainsbury's Stonebaked Margherita Pizza 10"	290	698.9	12.2	82.1	2.00
Gino's Minced Keema	320	780.8	12.2	81.6	1.50
Sainsbury's Classic Crust Tandoori Chicken Limited Edition	530	1213.7	12.2	161.1	3.00
Tesco Deep Pan Meat Feast	386	965.0	12.4	127.4	1.00
Tesco Stonebaked Thin Mediterranean Vegetable	390	760.5	12.5	106.5	1.50
Morrisons Meat Feast Crispy	313	845.1	12.5	104.5	2.00
Sainsbury's Thin & Crispy Cheese & Tomato Pizza 10"	265	736.7	12.7	78.2	1.80
Waitrose 1 Speck & Gorgonzola	295	873.2	12.7	101.5	4.89
Tesco Deep Pan Cheese	386	914.8	12.7	123.5	1.00

Suggested Brands	Size (g)	Kcal	S.fat (g)	Carbs (g)	£
Waitrose hand stretched ham & pineapple	410	1115.2	12.7	148.4	4.50
Pizza Express American	250	677.5	12.8	76.3	2.50
Morrisons The Best Sri Lankan Chicken	475	1135.3	12.8	151.5	4.00
Sainsbury's Deliciously Free From Vegan Margherita	330	716.1	12.9	99.7	3.50
Iceland Meat Feast Deep Pan Pizza	358	959.4	12.9	114.6	1.00
Morrisons Market St Takeaway Chicken & Bacon	560	1517.6	12.9	230.2	3.50
Morrisons Extra Thin Tex Mex	370	876.9	13.0	78.1	1.50
Sainsbury's Thin & Crispy Pepperoni	314	829.0	13.2	98.0	1.00
ASDA Spicy Meat Feast Thin Stonebaked 10"	290	719.2	13.3	84.1	1.87
Pizza Express American Hot	260	720.2	13.3	80.9	5.00
Morrisons V Taste Diced Tomato & Dried Basil Margherita	340	737.8	13.3	102.7	3.00
Sainsbury's Stonebaked Chargrilled Vegetable & Goats' Cheese	392	862.4	13.3	100.7	2.00
Crosta & Mollica Margherita Tomato, Mozzarella & Oregano Wood-Fired Sourdough	403	926.9	13.3	120.9	4.00

COMMON FOOD   PIZZA (WHOLE)

Suggested Brands	Size (g)	Kcal	S.fat (g)	Carbs (g)	£
Morrisons Thin & Crispy Cheese Feast	285	786.6	13.4	102.6	2.00
essential Waitrose cheese & tomato	300	870.0	13.5	98.1	1.40
Whole Creations Dairy & Gluten Free Roasted Tomato & Basil Sheesy	375	945.0	13.5	138.8	3.75
Goodfella's Pepperoni Thin Pizza	340	880.6	13.6	98.6	2.00
Sainsbury's Chicken Arrabiata With Nduja Pizza, Taste the Difference	470	1175.0	13.6	135.8	4.50
Sainsbury's Classic Crust Veggie Delight	565	1248.7	13.6	166.7	4.20
Morrisons Deep Pan Meat Feast	415	1050.0	13.7	140.3	1.00
Waitrose 1 wood-fired spicy calabrian salami	300	759.0	13.8	78.3	3.89
Sainsbury's Classic Crust BBQ Chicken	530	1340.9	13.8	177.6	4.20
Schar Lactose Free Margherita	280	644.0	14.0	75.6	3.00
Goodfella's Gluten Free Pepperoni, Ham & Mushroom	349	896.9	14.0	104.7	3.00
Iceland Stonebaked Spicy Double Pepperoni	370	854.7	14.1	105.5	1.59
Morrisons The Best Hoisin Pork	470	1109.2	14.1	145.2	4.00

COMMON FOOD PIZZA (WHOLE)

Suggested Brands	Size (g)	Kcal	S.fat (g)	Carbs (g)	£
Waitrose hand stretched garlic mushroom & spinach	395	1074.4	14.2	141.4	4.50
Sainsbury's Thin & Crispy Pepperoni Pizza 10'	275	775.5	14.3	75.9	2.00
Sainsbury's Stonebaked Pepperoni Pizza 10''	310	806.0	14.3	85.9	2.00
essential Waitrose thin & crispy pepperoni	255	762.5	14.5	77.8	2.50
Iceland Four Cheese Thin	322	821.1	14.5	83.7	1.00
ASDA Pepperoni Thin & Crispy Pizza	330	904.2	14.5	112.2	0.90
Morrisons Thin Pepperoni	346	961.9	14.5	115.2	1.00
Goodfella's Roast Chicken Stonebaked Thin Pizza	365	996.5	14.6	113.2	2.00
Sainsbury's Salami, Prosciutto & Chorizo Pizza, Taste the Difference	445	1134.8	14.7	132.6	4.50
Crosta & Mollica Piccante Spicy Salami, Rocket & Red Pepper Wood-Fired Sourdough Pizza	436	1042.0	14.8	126.4	4.00
Sainsbury's Deep Pan Meat Feast	402	1025.1	14.9	125.4	1.30
Morrisons Deep Pan Cheese	426	1052.2	14.9	142.7	1.00
Morrisons The Best Meat Feast	465	1190.4	14.9	151.6	4.00
Sainsbury's Thin & Crispy Meat Feast Pizza 10''	325	848.3	15.0	79.3	2.00

Suggested Brands	Size (g)	Kcal	S.fat (g)	Carbs (g)	£
Morrisons Triple Pepperoni Sourdough	333	869.1	15.0	94.9	1.50
Dr. Oetker Yes It's Pizza Beetroot Based Ham & Vegetable	315	743.4	15.1	78.8	3.00
Dr. Oetker Ristorante Mozzarella	335	861.0	15.1	7.0	2.50
Morrisons Deep Pan Pepperoni	398	1046.7	15.1	131.7	1.00
Morrisons The Best Cajun Chicken & Sweet Red Peppers	426	979.8	15.3	114.6	2.50
ASDA Cheese Feast Thin Stonebaked 10"	290	733.7	15.4	81.2	1.87
Dr. Oetker Ristorante Speciale	330	871.2	15.5	85.8	2.50
ASDA Meat Feast Deep Pan	400	1004.0	15.6	124.0	0.90
Waitrose hand stretched margherita	400	1088.0	15.6	132.0	4.50
Sainsbury's Thin & Crispy Cheese & Tomato	327	882.9	15.7	104.3	1.00
Waitrose 1 mozzarella & tomato	480	1281.6	15.8	165.1	5.59
Sainsbury's Deep Pan Pepperoni	401	1062.7	16.0	131.1	1.00
Morrisons Pepperoni Thin & Crispy	287	878.2	16.1	101.9	2.00
ASDA Pepperoni Thin Stonebaked 10"	289	754.3	16.2	75.1	1.87

COMMON FOOD   PIZZA (WHOLE)

Suggested Brands	Size (g)	Kcal	S.fat (g)	Carbs (g)	£
ASDA Double Pepperoni Deep Pan	386	1026.8	16.2	123.5	0.90
ASDA Extra Special Smoked Ham, Mushroom & Mascarpone 12"	392	956.5	16.5	98.0	3.59
Morrisons Meat Feast Sourdough	377	999.1	16.6	91.6	1.50
Sainsbury's Deliciously Free From Margherita	300	861.0	16.8	99.9	2.50
Goodfella's Pepperoni Deep Pan Baked	419	1068.5	16.8	15.1	2.00
Sainsbury's Stonebaked Roasted Tomato & Green Pesto	383	972.8	16.9	100.3	2.00
Tesco Stonebaked Thin Double Pepperoni	330	854.7	17.2	88.1	1.50
Morrisons The Best Margherita	465	1143.9	17.2	141.8	4.00
Iceland Double Pepperoni Deep Pan	385	1043.4	17.3	120.1	1.00
Sainsbury's Stonebaked Hot & Spicy Meat Feast	387	998.5	17.4	96.0	2.00
Sainsbury's Prosciutto Mushroom & Mascarpone Pizza, Taste the Difference	500	1170.0	17.5	131.5	4.50
Waitrose 1 wood-fired king prawn, garlic & chilli	500	1285.0	17.5	154.0	5.59
Sainsbury's Mozzarella & Cherry Tomato Pizza, Taste the Difference	490	1161.3	17.6	131.3	4.00

Suggested Brands	Size (g)	Kcal	S.fat (g)	Carbs (g)	£
Pizza Express Margherita 12"	455	1019.2	17.7	121.0	3.00
Sainsbury's Deep Pan Cheese & Tomato	403	1051.8	17.7	132.6	1.00
Sainsbury's Cheese & Tomato Pizza, Basics 12"	440	1236.4	18.0	153.6	1.60
Morrisons Stuffed Crust Cheese	420	1075.2	18.1	123.5	2.00
ASDA Stonebaked Double Pepperoni	364	961.0	18.2	101.9	1.20
Sainsbury's Deliciously Free From Pepperoni	300	987.0	18.3	89.7	2.50
Tesco Stonebaked Thin Four Cheese	330	828.3	18.5	89.8	1.50
Morrisons Takeaway Pulled Pork	547	1367.5	18.6	181.1	2.00
Iceland Double Pepperoni Thin	320	979.2	18.9	95.4	1.00
Sainsbury's Thin & Crispy Four Cheese	377	999.1	18.9	113.1	1.40
Pizza Express Sloppy Guiseppe 12 I	560	1187.2	19.0	148.4	3.00
Goodfella's Cheese Deep Pan Baked Pizza	417	1113.4	19.2	120.9	2.00
Sainsbury's Takeaway Stuffed Crust Pepperoni	424	1119.4	19.5	136.1	2.25
Morrisons The Best Ham, Mushroom & Mascarpone	515	1210.3	19.6	145.7	4.00
Sainsbury's Classic Crust Meat Feast	520	1326.0	19.8	150.3	3.00

Suggested Brands	Size (g)	Kcal	S.fat (g)	Carbs (g)	£
Morrisons Hot Dog Stuffed Crust	495	1336.5	19.8	153.0	2.00
ASDA 4 Cheese & Tomato Mini	356	1043.1	19.9	113.9	2.00
Sainsbury's Fig, Prosciutto Di Speck & Gorgonzola Pizza, Taste the Difference	445	1357.3	20.0	138.0	5.00
Waitrose hand stretched mushroom, bacon & mascarpone	440	1126.4	20.2	118.8	4.50
Iceland Stonebaked Sharing Margherita	450	1228.5	20.3	160.7	3.00
Iceland Four Cheese Deep Pan	408	1040.4	20.4	114.2	1.00
Goodfella's Margherita Thin Pizza	345	1028.1	20.7	110.4	2.00
Morrisons Market St Takeaway Meat Feast Pizza	560	1540.0	20.7	185.9	3.50
Pizza Express Margherita	245	600.3	20.8	77.2	2.50
Waitrose hand stretched pepperoni	385	1243.6	20.8	135.1	4.50
Sainsbury's Takeaway Fully Loaded BBQ Pulled Pork	547	1444.1	20.8	171.8	2.00
Iceland Cheese & Tomato Thin Sharing	510	1443.3	20.9	167.3	2.00
Morrisons Stuffed Crust Pepperoni	429	1154.0	21.0	119.7	2.00

COMMON FOOD   PIZZA (WHOLE)

Suggested Brands	Size (g)	Kcal	S.fat (g)	Carbs (g)	£
ASDA Four Cheese Deep Pan Pizza	407	1033.8	21.2	122.1	0.90
ASDA Four Cheese Deep Pan	407	1033.8	21.2	122.1	0.90
essential Waitrose cheese & tomato	500	1315.0	21.5	144.0	3.49
Sainsbury's Takeaway Fully Loaded Fiery Chicken	570	1413.6	22.2	153.9	2.00
Morrisons Stuffed Crust Cheese Feast	450	1228.5	22.5	141.8	3.50
Morrisons Takeaway Chicken & Bacon	535	1385.7	23.0	150.3	2.00
Iceland Takeaway Stuffed Crust Hot & Spicy Chicken	465	1162.5	23.3	138.1	2.00
Sainsbury's Takeaway Stuffed Crust Four Cheese	445	1179.3	24.0	138.8	2.25
Morrisons Best Four Cheese	416	1119.0	24.5	117.7	2.50
Morrisons Takeaway Tex Mex	553	1399.1	24.9	154.3	2.00
Morrisons The Best Spicy Milano Salami & 'Nduja	405	1121.9	25.1	110.2	2.50
Morrisons Take Away Stuffed Crust Pepperoni	467	1340.3	25.7	147.1	3.50
Iceland Pepperoni Sharing Thin	555	1581.8	26.6	166.5	2.00
Sainsbury's Takeaway Fully Loaded American Hot	542	1414.6	27.1	137.1	2.00

COMMON FOOD   PIZZA (WHOLE)

Suggested Brands	Size (g)	Kcal	S.fat (g)	Carbs (g)	£
Waitrose hand stretched feta & caramelised onion	440	1333.2	27.7	150.5	4.50
Iceland Takeaway Cheese Stuffed Crust Pepperoni	429	1261.3	27.9	148.4	2.00
Chicago Town The Pizza Kitchen Cheese Medley	350	1074.5	29.8	108.5	3.00
Chicago Town The Pizza Kitchen Pepperoni	355	1107.6	29.8	103.0	3.00
Iceland Takeaway Hot Dog Stuffed Crust New Yorker	551	1394.0	29.8	132.2	2.00
Iceland Meat Combo Classic Crust	790	1943.4	30.0	267.8	4.00
Iceland Takeaway Hot Dog Stuffed Crust Cheese & Tomato	531	1492.1	30.3	158.2	2.00
Sainsbury's Stuffed Crust Pepperoni Delight	620	1816.6	30.4	186.6	3.00
Sainsbury's Takeaway Fully Loaded Meat Feast	560	1596.0	30.8	153.4	2.00
Sainsbury's Stuffed Crust Cheese Feast	600	1746.0	31.2	190.8	3.00
Chicago Town Takeaway Large Chicken & Bacon Classic Crust	495	1430.6	31.7	158.4	4.00
Goodfella's Takeaway Mighty Meat	596	1740.3	34.0	166.9	3.00
Chicago Town The Pizza Kitchen Roasted Chicken	385	939.4	34.3	107.8	3.00
Iceland Takeaway Stuffed Crust Cheese Feast	453	1359.0	34.9	159.0	2.00

COMMON FOOD   PIZZA (WHOLE)

Suggested Brands	Size (g)	Kcal	S.fat (g)	Carbs (g)	£
Goodfella's Takeaway Big Cheese	555	1692.8	35.5	16.7	3.00
Goodfella's Takeaway Loaded Pepperoni	553	1764.1	39.8	138.3	3.00
Chicago Town Takeaway Large Pepperoni Stuffed Crust	645	1928.6	43.9	212.9	4.00
Chicago Town Takeaway Large Four Cheese Stuffed Crust	630	1839.6	44.1	207.9	4.00
Dr. Oetker Ristorante Pepperoni-Salame	320	899.2	44.8	16.0	1.50

SHOWS PER FULL PIZZA CONSUMED

Find Us On

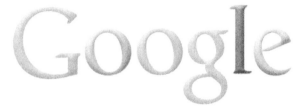

Search: **NADIET.INFO**

Pizza (Slice)

Suggested Brands	Size (g)	Kcal	S.fat (g)	Carbs (g)	£
ASDA Cheese & Ham Pizza	114	75.8	0.6	10.8	0.61
No Cheese Italian Garden	382	186.2	0.8	27.7	2.00
ASDA Cheese & Tomato Pizza	110	73.7	0.9	10.2	0.61
No Cheese Houmous	284	175.4	1.1	17.1	2.00
Sainsbury's Cheese & Tomato Pizza, Basics 7''	119	91.3	1.3	12.2	0.75
ASDA Smart Price Cheese & Tomato	268	156.8	1.4	23.5	0.60
Morrisons Sweet Chilli Chicken Extra Thin	362	247.1	1.5	30.0	1.50
Morrisons BBQ Chicken Sourdough	395	209.4	1.6	28.1	1.50
Pizza Express La Reine	290	153.0	1.7	20.1	5.00
Tesco Stonebaked Thin Sweet Chilli Chicken	330	184.8	1.8	24.9	1.50
Iceland Vegetable Thin	329	189.2	1.8	24.6	1.00
Morrisons 2 Pepperoni Pizza Baguettes	225	126.0	1.9	15.7	1.00
Pizza Express Vegan Giardiniera	272	137.4	2.0	20.6	5.00
Chicago Town 3 Cheese & Tomato Pizza Toasties	225	160.9	2.0	20.8	1.65
Iceland Southern Spiced Chicken Thin	336	210.0	2.0	25.6	1.00
Morrisons Ham & Pineapple Thin & Crispy	315	190.6	2.1	27.5	2.00

COMMON FOOD   PIZZA (SLICE)

Suggested Brands	Size (g)	Kcal	S.fat (g)	Carbs (g)	£
Iceland Chicken Fajita Thin	335	201.9	2.1	25.0	1.00
Iceland Barbecue Chicken Thin	334	213.8	2.1	28.0	1.00
Iceland Ham & Mushroom Deep Pan	413	225.1	2.1	33.3	1.00
Morrisons Spicy Chicken Thin & Crispy	320	183.2	2.2	24.7	2.00
Morrisons Cheese & Ham Thin	345	205.3	2.2	26.4	1.00
ASDA Cheese & Tomato (Margherita) Thin & Crispy Pizza	330	207.9	2.2	27.2	0.90
Tesco Stonebaked Thin Bbq Meat Feast	340	214.2	2.2	29.2	1.50
Morrisons The Best Chargrilled Vegetables	510	275.4	2.2	36.9	4.00
Whole Creations Butternut Squash, Red Pepper & Caramelised Onion Sheesy	300	146.3	2.3	22.4	3.75
Morrisons Mediterranean Veg Extra Thin	375	205.3	2.3	21.5	1.50
Iceland Ham & Pineapple Thin	345	206.2	2.3	26.5	1.00
Chicago Town 2 Deep Dish Chicken Club	320	208.8	2.3	25.6	2.00
Morrisons Mozzarella & Pesto Sourdough	353	225.1	2.3	27.5	1.50
Sainsbury's Deep Pan BBQ Chicken	422	247.9	2.3	37.1	1.30

Suggested Brands	Size (g)	Kcal	S.fat (g)	Carbs (g)	£
Hearty Food Thin Cheese And Tomato	314	197.0	2.4	27.9	0.67
ASDA Sweet Chilli Chicken Extra Thin & Crisp	375	202.5	2.4	22.5	1.20
Morrisons Thin Cheese	318	206.7	2.4	30.4	1.00
ASDA Fajita Chicken Stonebaked 10"	330	172.4	2.5	19.8	1.87
Sainsbury's Stonebaked Chicken & Pesto Pizza 10"	315	186.7	2.5	20.1	2.00
Iceland Stonebaked Mediterranean Vegetable	408	189.7	2.5	27.7	1.59
Waitrose 1 wood-fired buffalo mozzarella & sun soaked tomato	295	191.0	2.5	24.3	3.89
Iceland Stonebaked BBQ Chicken & Bacon	345	192.4	2.5	26.0	1.59
Iceland Stonebaked Sweet Chilli Chicken	415	202.3	2.5	29.6	1.59
Waitrose Vegan Stonebaked Margherita	385	210.8	2.5	33.1	4.99
Sainsbury's Thin & Crispy Hawaiian	413	221.0	2.5	30.4	1.40
ASDA Cheese & Tomato 10"	257	174.1	2.6	21.9	1.11
Sainsbury's Stonebaked Spinach & Ricotta Pizza 10'	320	181.6	2.6	22.8	3.00
Waitrose 1 wood-fired roasted vegetable & pesto	335	198.5	2.6	25.1	3.89

Suggested Brands	Size (g)	Kcal	S.fat (g)	Carbs (g)	£
Tesco Stonebaked Ham And Pineapple	375	205.3	2.6	25.0	1.50
ASDA Mediterranean Vegetable Extra Thin & Crispy	375	238.1	2.6	5.4	1.20
Dr. Oetker Yes It's Pizza Spinach Based Broccoli & Mushroom	335	174.2	2.7	18.4	3.00
Hearty Food Thin Pepperoni	314	203.3	2.7	25.8	0.67
Sainsbury's Vegetable	406	219.3	2.7	28.6	1.40
Goodfella's Romano Chicken, Roquito Pepper & Red Onion with a Garlic Oil Drizzle	389	229.5	2.7	25.3	2.50
Iceland Double Cheeseburger Deep Pan	380	250.8	2.7	34.7	1.00
Waitrose hand stretched pepper & ricotta	430	263.4	2.7	36.9	4.50
Morrisons Savers Cheese & Tomato	220	141.9	2.8	17.1	0.95
Sainsbury's Stonebaked Ham & Pineapple Pizza 10"	305	180.0	2.8	21.8	2.00
Dr. Oetker Ristorante Thin & Crispy Pollo	355	197.9	2.8	23.1	2.50
Goodfella's Ham & Pineapple Thin	365	210.8	2.8	26.5	2.00
Sainsbury's Spicy Chicken	404	227.3	2.8	29.4	1.40

Suggested Brands	Size (g)	Kcal	S.fat (g)	Carbs (g)	£
Iceland Chicken & Sweetcorn Pizza Deep Pan	411	238.4	2.8	31.5	1.00
Sainsbury's Stonebaked Hot & Spicy Pizza 10''	320	180.8	2.9	20.3	3.00
Iceland Cheese & Ham Thin	327	214.2	2.9	25.0	1.00
ASDA Stonebaked BBQ Chicken	395	224.2	2.9	28.7	1.20
Waitrose hand stretched chicken & chorizo	395	262.7	2.9	31.6	4.50
The White Rabbit Pizza Co. Smokin' Vegan	340	185.3	3.0	26.6	5.00
ASDA BBQ Chicken Deep Pan Pizza	423	242.2	3.0	33.9	0.90
Sainsbury's Stonebaked Margherita Pizza 10''	290	174.7	3.1	20.5	2.00
Tesco Stonebaked Thin Mediterranean Vegetable	390	190.1	3.1	26.6	1.50
Gino's Minced Keema	320	195.2	3.1	20.4	1.50
Morrisons Meat Feast Crispy	313	211.3	3.1	26.1	2.00
Tesco Deep Pan Meat Feast	386	241.3	3.1	31.9	1.00
Sainsbury's Classic Crust Tandoori Chicken Limited Edition	530	303.4	3.1	40.3	3.00
Pizza Express American	250	169.4	3.2	19.1	2.50
Sainsbury's Deliciously Free From Vegan Margherita	330	179.0	3.2	24.9	3.50

Suggested Brands	Size (g)	Kcal	S.fat (g)	Carbs (g)	£
Sainsbury's Thin & Crispy Cheese & Tomato Pizza 10"	265	184.2	3.2	19.6	1.80
Waitrose 1 Speck & Gorgonzola	295	218.3	3.2	25.4	4.89
Tesco Deep Pan Cheese	386	228.7	3.2	30.9	1.00
Iceland Meat Feast Deep Pan Pizza	358	239.9	3.2	28.7	1.00
Waitrose hand stretched ham & pineapple	410	278.8	3.2	37.1	4.50
Morrisons The Best Sri Lankan Chicken	475	283.8	3.2	37.9	4.00
Morrisons Market St Takeaway Chicken & Bacon	560	379.4	3.2	57.6	3.50
ASDA Spicy Meat Feast Thin Stonebaked 10"	290	179.8	3.3	21.0	1.87
Pizza Express American Hot	260	180.1	3.3	20.2	5.00
Morrisons V Taste Diced Tomato & Dried Basil Margherita	340	184.5	3.3	25.7	3.00
Sainsbury's Thin & Crispy Pepperoni	314	207.3	3.3	24.5	1.00
Sainsbury's Stonebaked Chargrilled Vegetable & Goats' Cheese	392	215.6	3.3	25.2	2.00
Morrisons Extra Thin Tex Mex	370	219.2	3.3	19.5	1.50
Crosta & Mollica Margherita Tomato,	403	231.7	3.3	30.2	4.00

Suggested Brands	Size (g)	Kcal	S.fat (g)	Carbs (g)	£
Mozzarella & Oregano Wood-Fired Sourdough					
Morrisons Thin & Crispy Cheese Feast	285	196.7	3.4	25.7	2.00
essential Waitrose cheese & tomato	300	217.5	3.4	24.5	1.40
Goodfella's Pepperoni Thin Pizza	340	220.2	3.4	24.7	2.00
Whole Creations Dairy & Gluten Free Roasted Tomato & Basil Sheesy	375	236.3	3.4	34.7	3.75
Morrisons Deep Pan Meat Feast	415	262.5	3.4	35.1	1.00
Sainsbury's Chicken Arrabiata With Nduja Pizza, Taste the Difference	470	293.8	3.4	34.0	4.50
Sainsbury's Classic Crust Veggie Delight	565	312.2	3.4	41.7	4.20
Schar Lactose Free Margherita	280	161.0	3.5	18.9	3.00
Waitrose 1 wood-fired spicy calabrian salami	300	189.8	3.5	19.6	3.89
Iceland Stonebaked Spicy Double Pepperoni	370	213.7	3.5	26.4	1.59
Goodfella's Gluten Free Pepperoni, Ham & Mushroom	349	224.2	3.5	26.2	3.00
Morrisons The Best Hoisin Pork	470	277.3	3.5	36.3	4.00

COMMON FOOD   PIZZA (SLICE)

Suggested Brands	Size (g)	Kcal	S.fat (g)	Carbs (g)	£
Sainsbury's Classic Crust BBQ Chicken	530	335.2	3.5	44.4	4.20
essential Waitrose thin & crispy pepperoni	255	190.6	3.6	19.5	2.50
Sainsbury's Thin & Crispy Pepperoni Pizza 10'	275	193.9	3.6	19.0	2.00
Sainsbury's Stonebaked Pepperoni Pizza 10''	310	201.5	3.6	21.5	2.00
Iceland Four Cheese Thin	322	205.3	3.6	20.9	1.00
ASDA Pepperoni Thin & Crispy Pizza	330	226.1	3.6	28.1	0.90
Morrisons Thin Pepperoni	346	240.5	3.6	28.8	1.00
Waitrose hand stretched garlic mushroom & spinach	395	268.6	3.6	35.4	4.50
Goodfella's Roast Chicken Stonebaked Thin Pizza	365	249.1	3.7	28.3	2.00
Sainsbury's Deep Pan Meat Feast	402	256.3	3.7	31.4	1.30
Crosta & Mollica Piccante Spicy Salami, Rocket & Red Pepper Wood-Fired Sourdough Pizza	436	260.5	3.7	31.6	4.00
Morrisons Deep Pan Cheese	426	263.1	3.7	35.7	1.00
Sainsbury's Salami, Prosciutto & Chorizo Pizza, Taste the Difference	445	283.7	3.7	33.2	4.50
Morrisons The Best Meat Feast	465	297.6	3.7	37.9	4.00

Suggested Brands	Size (g)	Kcal	S.fat (g)	Carbs (g)	£
Dr. Oetker Yes It's Pizza Beetroot Based Ham & Vegetable	315	185.9	3.8	19.7	3.00
Sainsbury's Thin & Crispy Meat Feast Pizza 10"	325	212.1	3.8	19.8	2.00
Dr. Oetker Ristorante Mozzarella	335	215.3	3.8	1.8	2.50
Morrisons Triple Pepperoni Sourdough	333	217.3	3.8	23.7	1.50
Morrisons The Best Cajun Chicken & Sweet Red Peppers	426	245.0	3.8	28.7	2.50
Morrisons Deep Pan Pepperoni	398	261.7	3.8	32.9	1.00
ASDA Cheese Feast Thin Stonebaked 10"	290	183.4	3.9	20.3	1.87
Dr. Oetker Ristorante Speciale	330	217.8	3.9	21.5	2.50
Sainsbury's Thin & Crispy Cheese & Tomato	327	220.7	3.9	26.1	1.00
ASDA Meat Feast Deep Pan	400	251.0	3.9	31.0	0.90
Waitrose hand stretched margherita	400	272.0	3.9	33.0	4.50
Morrisons Pepperoni Thin & Crispy	287	219.6	4.0	25.5	2.00
Sainsbury's Deep Pan Pepperoni	401	265.7	4.0	32.8	1.00
Waitrose 1 mozzarella & tomato	480	320.4	4.0	41.3	5.59

Suggested Brands	Size (g)	Kcal	S.fat (g)	Carbs (g)	£
ASDA Pepperoni Thin Stonebaked 10"	289	188.6	4.1	18.8	1.87
ASDA Extra Special Smoked Ham, Mushroom & Mascarpone 12"	392	239.1	4.1	24.5	3.59
ASDA Double Pepperoni Deep Pan	386	256.7	4.1	30.9	0.90
Sainsbury's Deliciously Free From Margherita	300	215.3	4.2	25.0	2.50
Sainsbury's Stonebaked Roasted Tomato & Green Pesto	383	243.2	4.2	25.1	2.00
Morrisons Meat Feast Sourdough	377	249.8	4.2	22.9	1.50
Goodfella's Pepperoni Deep Pan Baked	419	267.1	4.2	3.8	2.00
Tesco Stonebaked Thin Double Pepperoni	330	213.7	4.3	22.0	1.50
Iceland Double Pepperoni Deep Pan	385	260.9	4.3	30.0	1.00
Morrisons The Best Margherita	465	286.0	4.3	35.5	4.00
Sainsbury's Stonebaked Hot & Spicy Meat Feast	387	249.6	4.4	24.0	2.00
Pizza Express Margherita 12"	455	254.8	4.4	30.3	3.00
Sainsbury's Deep Pan Cheese & Tomato	403	263.0	4.4	33.2	1.00
Sainsbury's Mozzarella & Cherry Tomato Pizza, Taste the Difference	490	290.3	4.4	32.8	4.00

Suggested Brands	Size (g)	Kcal	S.fat (g)	Carbs (g)	£
Sainsbury's Prosciutto Mushroom & Mascarpone Pizza, Taste the Difference	500	292.5	4.4	32.9	4.50
Waitrose 1 wood-fired king prawn, garlic & chilli	500	321.3	4.4	38.5	5.59
Morrisons Stuffed Crust Cheese	420	268.8	4.5	30.9	2.00
Sainsbury's Cheese & Tomato Pizza, Basics 12''	440	309.1	4.5	38.4	1.60
Tesco Stonebaked Thin Four Cheese	330	207.1	4.6	22.5	1.50
ASDA Stonebaked Double Pepperoni	364	240.3	4.6	25.5	1.20
Sainsbury's Deliciously Free From Pepperoni	300	246.8	4.6	22.4	2.50
Iceland Double Pepperoni Thin	320	244.8	4.7	23.9	1.00
Sainsbury's Thin & Crispy Four Cheese	377	249.8	4.7	28.3	1.40
Morrisons Takeaway Pulled Pork	547	341.9	4.7	45.3	2.00
Goodfella's Cheese Deep Pan Baked Pizza	417	278.4	4.8	30.2	2.00
Pizza Express Sloppy Guiseppe 12 I	560	296.8	4.8	37.1	3.00
Sainsbury's Takeaway Stuffed Crust Pepperoni	424	279.9	4.9	34.0	2.25
Morrisons The Best Ham, Mushroom & Mascarpone	515	302.6	4.9	36.4	4.00

Suggested Brands	Size (g)	Kcal	S.fat (g)	Carbs (g)	£
ASDA 4 Cheese & Tomato Mini	356	260.8	5.0	28.5	2.00
Sainsbury's Classic Crust Meat Feast	520	331.5	5.0	37.6	3.00
Morrisons Hot Dog Stuffed Crust	495	334.1	5.0	38.3	2.00
Sainsbury's Fig, Prosciutto Di Speck & Gorgonzola Pizza, Taste the Difference	445	339.3	5.0	34.5	5.00
Iceland Four Cheese Deep Pan	408	260.1	5.1	28.6	1.00
Waitrose hand stretched mushroom, bacon & mascarpone	440	281.6	5.1	29.7	4.50
Iceland Stonebaked Sharing Margherita	450	307.1	5.1	40.2	3.00
Pizza Express Margherita	245	150.1	5.2	19.3	2.50
Goodfella's Margherita Thin Pizza	345	257.0	5.2	27.6	2.00
Waitrose hand stretched pepperoni	385	310.9	5.2	33.8	4.50
Iceland Cheese & Tomato Thin Sharing	510	360.8	5.2	41.8	2.00
Sainsbury's Takeaway Fully Loaded BBQ Pulled Pork	547	361.0	5.2	43.0	2.00
Morrisons Market St Takeaway Meat Feast Pizza	560	385.0	5.2	46.5	3.50

COMMON FOOD PIZZA (SLICE)

Suggested Brands	Size (g)	Kcal	S.fat (g)	Carbs (g)	£
ASDA Four Cheese Deep Pan Pizza	407	258.5	5.3	30.5	0.90
ASDA Four Cheese Deep Pan	407	258.5	5.3	30.5	0.90
Morrisons Stuffed Crust Pepperoni	429	288.5	5.3	29.9	2.00
essential Waitrose cheese & tomato	500	328.8	5.4	36.0	3.49
Morrisons Stuffed Crust Cheese Feast	450	307.1	5.6	35.5	3.50
Sainsbury's Takeaway Fully Loaded Fiery Chicken	570	353.4	5.6	38.5	2.00
Iceland Takeaway Stuffed Crust Hot & Spicy Chicken	465	290.6	5.8	34.5	2.00
Morrisons Takeaway Chicken & Bacon	535	346.4	5.8	37.6	2.00
Sainsbury's Takeaway Stuffed Crust Four Cheese	445	294.8	6.0	34.7	2.25
Morrisons Best Four Cheese	416	279.8	6.1	29.4	2.50
Morrisons Takeaway Tex Mex	553	349.8	6.2	38.6	2.00
Morrisons The Best Spicy Milano Salami & 'Nduja	405	280.5	6.3	27.6	2.50
Morrisons Take Away Stuffed Crust Pepperoni	467	335.1	6.4	36.8	3.50
Iceland Pepperoni Sharing Thin	555	395.5	6.7	41.6	2.00

COMMON FOOD   PIZZA (SLICE)

Suggested Brands	Size (g)	Kcal	S.fat (g)	Carbs (g)	£
Sainsbury's Takeaway Fully Loaded American Hot	542	353.7	6.8	34.3	2.00
Waitrose hand stretched feta & caramelised onion	440	333.3	6.9	37.6	4.50
Iceland Takeaway Cheese Stuffed Crust Pepperoni	429	315.3	7.0	37.1	2.00
Chicago Town The Pizza Kitchen Cheese Medley	350	268.6	7.5	27.1	3.00
Chicago Town The Pizza Kitchen Pepperoni	355	276.9	7.5	25.8	3.00
Iceland Takeaway Hot Dog Stuffed Crust New Yorker	551	348.5	7.5	33.1	2.00
Iceland Meat Combo Classic Crust	790	485.9	7.5	67.0	4.00
Iceland Takeaway Hot Dog Stuffed Crust Cheese & Tomato	531	373.0	7.6	39.6	2.00
Sainsbury's Stuffed Crust Pepperoni Delight	620	454.2	7.6	46.7	3.00
Sainsbury's Takeaway Fully Loaded Meat Feast	560	399.0	7.7	38.4	2.00
Sainsbury's Stuffed Crust Cheese Feast	600	436.5	7.8	47.7	3.00
Chicago Town Takeaway Large Chicken & Bacon Classic Crust	495	357.7	7.9	39.6	4.00
Goodfella's Takeaway Mighty Meat	596	435.1	8.5	41.7	3.00

COMMON FOOD PIZZA (SLICE)

Suggested Brands	Size (g)	Kcal	S.fat (g)	Carbs (g)	£
Chicago Town The Pizza Kitchen Roasted Chicken	385	234.9	8.6	27.0	3.00
Iceland Takeaway Stuffed Crust Cheese Feast	453	339.8	8.7	39.8	2.00
Goodfella's Takeaway Big Cheese	555	423.2	8.9	4.2	3.00
Goodfella's Takeaway Loaded Pepperoni	553	441.0	10.0	34.6	3.00
Chicago Town Takeaway Large Four Cheese Stuffed Crust	630	459.9	11.0	52.0	4.00
Chicago Town Takeaway Large Pepperoni Stuffed Crust	645	482.2	11.0	53.2	4.00
Dr. Oetker Ristorante Pepperoni-Salame	320	224.8	11.2	4.0	1.50

SHOWS PER ¼ SLICE PIZZA CONSUMED

Rice

Suggested Brands	Size (g)	Kcal	S.fat (g)	Carbs (g)	£
Iceland 6 White Rice Steam Bags 1.2Kg	1200	136	0.0	31.1	1.89
Uncle Ben's Long Grain	1000	154	0.0	33.7	2.98
Uncle Ben's Boil in the Bag Long Grain	1000	154	0.0	33.7	4.98
Royal Umbrella Thai Jasmine	1000	347	0.0	81.6	2.10
Amira superior aromatic	1000	354	0.0	78.5	4.75
Amira pure basmati	1000	358	0.0	79.5	4.79
Morrisons Steam & Serve Riced Cauliflower	600	35	0.1	4.4	1.75
Veetee Extra Long Basmati	1000	84	0.1	18.2	3.50
ASDA 2 Steam Bags Mediterranean Vegetabl	400	88	0.1	16	1.25
orrisons 4 White Rice with Mixed Vegetables	600	100	0.1	19.4	1.75
Iceland 4 White Rice Steam Bags with Wild Rice & Vegetables	500	106	0.1	19.6	2.00
Veetee Thai Jasmine Rice	1000	109	0.1	24.7	3.50
Tesco 4 Steam Bags Rice With Mixed Vegetables	600	111	0.1	20.9	1.75
Morrisons Easy Cook Long Grain	1000	114	0.1	24.6	1.20
ASDA Boil in the Bag Long Grain White	1000	115	0.1	25	1.37
Morrisons Easy Cook Basmati	1000	115	0.1	24.7	1.60
Veetee Long Grain Rice	1000	116	0.1	26.6	2.50

COMMON FOOD   RICE

Suggested Brands	Size (g)	Kcal	S.fat (g)	Carbs (g)	£
Sainsbury's Easy Cook Long Grain	1000	117	0.1	25.1	1.20
Sainsbury's Long Grain	1000	117	0.1	25.4	1.20
Morrisons Basmati Rice	1000	117	0.1	25.1	1.67
essential Waitrose Basmati	1000	117	0.1	25.3	1.75
Sainsbury's Basmati Rice	1000	117	0.1	25.4	1.80
Waitrose Jasmine Hom Mali	1000	117	0.1	25.5	1.94
Waitrose basmati aromatic	1000	117	0.1	25.3	2.16
Sainsbury's Aged Indian Basmati Rice	1000	117	0.1	25.4	2.75
Sainsbury's White Rice, Basics	1000	119	0.1	25.8	0.45
Iceland 4 Golden Savoury Rice Steam Bags	600	120	0.1	21.4	2.00
Tesco Micro Rice Mexican Inspired	600	130	0.1	25.5	1.75
Sainsbury's White Rice Microwavable Bags x4	800	140	0.1	31.1	1.50
ASDA 4 Steam Bags Long Grain	800	140	0.1	31	1.75
Morrisons 4 White Rice	800	140	0.1	31.1	1.75
ASDA Long Grain White	1000	141	0.1	31	1.49
Tesco Micro Rice Long Grain White Rice 4 X 200G	800	144	0.1	31.5	1.75
ASDA Easy Cook Basmati White Rice	1000	145	0.1	32	1.44
Grower Harvest Long Grain	1000	153	0.1	33.1	0.45

Suggested Brands	Size (g)	Kcal	S.fat (g)	Carbs (g)	£
essential Waitrose easy cook long grain	1000	156	0.1	34.7	1.25
essential Waitrose long grain	1000	156	0.1	34.7	1.25
essential Waitrose white rice x 4 bags	720	156	0.1	34.7	1.40
ASDA Easy Cook Long Grain White	1000	158	0.1	35	0.94
Waitrose basmati & wild	1000	343	0.1	74.3	4.00
Bodrum Tosya Rice	1000	364	0.1	78.9	2.09
ASDA 2 Steam Bags Cauliflower Rice	400	33	0.2	3.5	1.25
Sainsbury's Rice, Broccoli, Sweetcorn & Peas Microwaveable Steam Bags x4	540	104	0.2	17.9	1.50
Sainsbury's Steamed Golden	380	111	0.2	21	1.20
Sainsbury's Steamed Mediterranean Vegetable	380	116	0.2	23	1.10
ASDA 2 Steam Bags Spicy Vegetable	400	119	0.2	22	1.25
Sainsbury's Brown Rice	1000	119	0.2	22.6	1.70
ASDA 2 Steam Bags Golden Vegetable	400	126	0.2	22	1.25
ASDA White Basmati Rice	1000	127	0.2	27	1.44
Tesco Micro Rice Egg Fried	600	135	0.2	26.2	1.75
ASDA 4 Steam Bags Wholegrain	800	141	0.2	29	1.50
Morrisons 4 Wholegrain Rice	600	142	0.2	29.2	1.75

Suggested Brands	Size (g)	Kcal	S.fat (g)	Carbs (g)	£
Tesco 4 Steam Bags Whole Grain	600	149	0.2	30.7	1.75
Iceland Takeaway Pilau	350	173	0.2	33.5	1.00
Tesco Arborio Risotto	1000	347	0.2	77.2	2.00
Akash Basmati Rice	1000	351	0.2	78.6	1.50
Tilda Pure Basmati	1000	351	0.2	77.7	4.99
Tesco Basmati	1000	356	0.2	77.4	1.60
Tesco 4 Steam Bags Vegetable With Fragrant Couscous	640	96	0.3	12.5	2.00
Birds Eye 2 Steamfresh Aromatic Indian	380	105	0.3	18	1.75
Birds Eye 2 Steamfresh Golden Vegetable	380	107	0.3	20	2.00
Morrisons Easy Cook Brown Long Grain	1000	110	0.3	19.3	1.83
Morrisons Brown Basmati	1000	114	0.3	20.8	1.70
Waitrose Duchy Organic whole grain	1000	119	0.3	22.5	3.29
Waitrose LOVE life basmati brown	1000	122	0.3	22.8	3.05
Tesco Chickpea Bulgur Wheat And Mixed Vegetables	600	130	0.3	21	2.00
ASDA 2 Steam Bags Egg Fried Rice with Peas	400	132	0.3	25	1.25
Veetee Brown Basmati	1000	138	0.3	28.9	3.00
ASDA Easy Cook Long Grain Brown Rice	1000	142	0.3	29	1.09
ASDA Long Grain Brown	1000	142	0.3	29	1.49
ASDA Brown Basmati	1000	165	0.3	33	1.77

Common Food   Rice

Suggested Brands	Size (g)	Kcal	S.fat (g)	Carbs (g)	£
ASDA Smart Price Long Grain Rice	1000	171	0.3	34	0.45
Tesco Finest Basmati	1000	349	0.3	76	3.00
Tesco Thai Fragrant Long Grain	1000	352	0.3	77.3	2.00
Tesco Easy Cook Long Grain	1000	353	0.3	78	1.20
Arirang Sushi Rice	1000	360	0.3	82	3.11
Iceland 4 Cauliflower Rice Steam Bags	600	45	0.4	3.0	2.00
Birds Eye 2 Steamfresh Mediterranean Vegetable	380	115	0.4	20	2.00
Sainsbury's Steamed Egg Fried	380	122	0.4	22	1.10
Uncle Bens Microwave Tomato and Basil	250	168	0.4	30.4	1.00
Iceland Takeaway Special Fried Rice	350	183	0.6	24.4	1.59
Iceland Takeaway Egg Fried	350	219	0.6	29.5	1.00
Tilda Wholegrain Basmati	1000	351	0.6	71.2	4.99
Tesco Easy Cook Brown	1000	356	0.6	74	1.50
ASDA 2 Steam Bags Green Vegetable Rice with a Herb Butter	400	106	1.5	17	1.25
Birds Eye 2 Steamfresh Tender Green Vegetable	380	114	2.1	17	2.00
Morrisons Pea & Spinach Risotto	500	202	2.2	32	1.75

Values Shown Per 100 Grams Uncooked

Sauces (BBQ)

Suggested Brands	Size (g)	Kcal	S.fat (g)	Carbs (g)	£
Skinny Smokey BBQ	425ml	4.5	0.0	0.5	3.99
Crucials BBQ Marinade Sauce	500ml	27.0	0.0	6.4	1.00
ASDA Smoky BBQ Marinade & Sauce	280	27.9	0.0	6.3	1.00
Morrisons Bourbon BBQ Sauce	295	28.8	0.0	6.3	1.00
Tesco Top Down Squeezy BBQ Sauce	480	33.6	0.0	7.8	1.00
ASDA Classic BBQ Sauce	460	37.5	0.0	9.0	1.00
HP Classic BBQ Sauce	465	39.9	0.0	9.5	1.50
Red's Kansas City BBQ Sauce Mild	300ml	39.9	0.0	9.1	1.99
Levi Roots Reggae Reggae Jerk BBQ Sauce	290	41.1	0.0	9.9	1.49
Sainsbury's Spicy BBQ Sauce	500	42.0	0.0	9.9	1.20
Hellmann's Smokey BBQ Sauce	430ml	42.3	0.0	8.7	2.00
Sainsbury's BBQ Sauce	500	43.5	0.0	10.1	1.20
Bull's-Eye Original BBQ Sauce	355	48.0	0.0	11.4	1.50
Jack Daniel's Smooth Original Barbecue Sauce	260	48.6	0.0	11.6	1.99
Tesco Reduced Salt & Sugar Bbq Sauce	470	27.6	0.1	6.0	1.00
Heinz Korean Style Sticky BBQ Sauce	220 ml	52.2	0.1	11.7	1.50

VALUES SHOWN PER 30 GRAMS SERVING

Sauces (Brown Sauce)

Suggested Brands	Size (g)	Kcal	S.fat (g)	Carbs (g)	£
Sainsbury's Brown Sauce, Reduced Salt & Sugar	450	21.9	0.0	4.9	0.90
Sainsbury's Brown Sauce, Basics	450	22.5	0.0	5.2	0.40
HP Expertly Blended Reduced Salt & Sugar Sauce	450	25.8	0.0	5.9	1.50
ASDA Brown Sauce	540	26.7	0.0	6.0	0.38
Daddies Favourite Brown Sauce	685	28.5	0.0	6.3	1.85
Tesco Squeezy Top Down Fruity Brown Sauce	480	30.3	0.0	6.8	0.90
ASDA Brown Sauce	480	32.1	0.0	7.2	0.55
essential Waitrose squeezy brown sauce	480	33.6	0.0	7.8	0.96
HP Brown Sauce	450	36.6	0.0	8.5	1.50
Chef Brown Sauce	485	36.6	0.0	9.0	1.50
HP Fruity Brown Sauce	470	40.5	0.0	9.5	1.50
Stokes Real Brown Sauce	320	48.6	0.0	11.6	2.99
Tesco Reduced Sugar & Salt Brown Sauce	460	26.4	0.1	5.1	0.90
Sainsbury's Brown Sauce	450	28.8	0.1	6.5	0.90
Tesco Squeezy Top Down Brown Sauce	480	31.2	0.1	6.3	0.90
Morrisons Squeezy Brown Sauce	470	31.5	0.1	6.8	1.00

VALUES SHOWN PER 30 GRAMS SERVING

Sauces (Chilli)

Suggested Brands	Size (g)	Kcal	S.fat (g)	Carbs (g)	£
Cholula Original Hot Sauce	150ml	5.7	0.0	0.1	1.79
Frank's RedHot Original Cayenne Pepper Sauce	148ml	7.5	0.0	0.5	1.49
Blue Dragon Thai Hot Chilli Sriracha Sauce	435ml	26.2	0.0	5.6	2.00
Blue Dragon Light Sweet Chilli Sauce	350	40.5	0.0	9.9	1.99
Tesco Sweet Chilli Dipping Sauce	290	48.9	0.0	11.8	1.25
Blue Dragon Mild Sweet Chilli Sauce	380	54.0	0.0	13.1	1.99
Blue Dragon Hot Sweet Chilli Sauce	380	55.2	0.0	13.1	1.99
Blue Dragon Original Sweet Chilli Sauce	380	55.2	0.0	13.1	1.99
Heinz Moreish & Tangy Sweet Chilli Sauce	220ml	55.5	0.0	13.8	1.50
Sainsbury's Sweet Chilli Sauce	300	58.5	0.0	14.4	1.25
ASDA Jalapeño Chilli Sauce	155ml	10.3	0.1	1.5	0.94
Crucials Extra Hot Chilli Sauce	500ml	13.5	0.1	1.9	1.00
Tesco Sriracha Hot Chilli Sauce	285	27.0	0.1	5.6	1.75
Hellmann's Garlic and Chilli Sauce	250ml	80.1	0.9	2.6	1.69

VALUES SHOWN PER 30 GRAMS SERVING

Sauces (Kebab, Curry, Burger and Bacon)

Suggested Brands	Size (g)	Kcal	S.fat (g)	Carbs (g)	£
Skinny Chip shop Curry	425ml	4.5	0.1	0.6	3.99
ASDA Chunky Burger Sauce	275	53.4	0.3	1.9	0.84
Sainsbury's Burger Sauce	300	58.5	0.4	3.2	1.20
Tesco Burger Sauce	250ml	62.4	0.5	3.0	1.00
Hellmann's Garlic Kebab Sauce	250ml	79.8	0.6	2.6	1.69
Heinz Burger Sauce	220ml	112.5	0.9	3.6	1.50
Heinz American Style Smokey Baconnaise Sauce	220ml	149.1	2.5	1.7	1.69

VALUES SHOWN PER 30 GRAMS SERVING

Sauces (Tomato Ketchup)

Suggested Brands	Size (g)	Kcal	S.fat (g)	Carbs (g)	£
Skinny Tomato Ketchup	425ml	6.2	0.0	1.1	3.99
ASDA Tomato Ketchup No Added Sugar & Salt	680	14.4	0.0	2.7	0.67
ASDA Tomato Ketchup 50% Reduced Sugar & Salt	700	18.9	0.0	3.9	0.67
Heinz Tomato Ketchup 50% Less Sugar & Salt	625	19.2	0.0	3.6	2.00
Morrisons Reduced Sugar & Salt Tomato Ketchup	465	20.1	0.0	4.1	0.80
Sainsbury's Tomato Ketchup, Reduced Salt	445	20.4	0.0	3.9	0.60
Sainsbury's Tomato Ketchup	460	28.5	0.0	6.0	0.60
Morrisons Squeezy Tomato Ketchup	470	28.5	0.0	6.5	0.80
Sainsbury's Tomato Ketchup, SO Organic	460	29.4	0.0	6.6	1.50
Heinz Tomato "Edchup" Ketchup	460	30.6	0.0	7.0	1.50
Heinz Tomato Ketchup	650	30.6	0.0	7.0	2.00
Sainsbury's Tomato Ketchup, Basics	460	30.6	0.0	7.0	0.45
ASDA Classic Tomato Ketchup	720	33.3	0.0	7.5	0.67
Daddies Tomato Ketchup	685	33.3	0.0	8.1	1.85
ASDA Tomato Ketchup (Smart Price)	500	34.5	0.0	8.1	0.40
Osem Kosher Ketchup	750	34.5	0.0	8.2	2.78

COMMON FOOD   SAUCES (TOMATO KETCHUP)

Suggested Brands	Size (g)	Kcal	S.fat (g)	Carbs (g)	£
Chef Squeezy Tomato Ketchup	490	37.5	0.0	8.7	1.50
Pudliszki Mild Ketchup	480	44.4	0.0	10.5	1.25
Tesco Top Down Tomato Ketchup Reduced Sugar And Salt	525	17.4	0.1	3.4	0.65
Tesco Top Down Tomato Ketchup	550	31.5	0.1	7.1	0.65
Tesco Organic Tomato Ketchup	460	33.3	0.2	6.9	1.50
Heinz Tomato Ketchup No Added Sugar & Salt	425	13.5	2.7	1.7	1.50

VALUES SHOWN PER 30 GRAMS SERVING

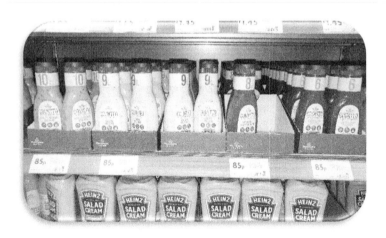

Sauces (Mayonnaise)

Suggested Brands	Size (g)	Kcal	S.fat (g)	Carbs (g)	£
Skinny Garlic And Herb	425ml	3.0	0.0	0.5	3.99
Sainsbury's Mayonnaise Squeezy, Be Good To Yourself	430ml	27.0	0.2	3.6	1.00
Asda Smart Price Mayonnaise	500g	81.6	0.6	3.0	0.41
Asda Light Mayonnaise	400ml	85.8	0.6	1.9	0.56
Sainsbury's Mayonnaise, Basics	500ml	90.3	0.6	3.9	0.55
Essential Waitrose Half Fat Mayonnaise	250ml	92.1	0.6	3.0	0.66
Nando's Perinaise Peri-Peri Mayonnaise Mild	265	92.7	0.6	3.9	1.50
Sainsbury's Reduced Fat Mayonnaise	730ml	77.7	0.7	2.0	1.20
Asda Garlic Mayonnaise	252	81.9	0.7	2.6	0.69
Tesco Light Mayonnaise	450ml	85.5	0.7	3.1	0.75
Nando's Perinaise Peri-Peri Hot Mayonnaise	265	98.1	0.7	4.2	1.50
Hellmann's Light Mayonnaise	600	79.2	0.8	1.8	2.00
Hellmann's Garlic Mayonnaise	235	80.1	0.8	2.0	1.00
Heinz Seriously Good Light Mayonnaise	720g	80.1	0.8	2.4	2.00
Tesco Reduced Calorie Light Mayonnaise	650ml	92.4	0.8	3.3	1.05
Tesco Garlic Mayonnaise	250ml	99.1	0.8	3.6	1.05

COMMON FOOD   SAUCES (MAYONNAISE)

Suggested Brands	Size (g)	Kcal	S.fat (g)	Carbs (g)	£
Crucials Garlic & Herb Sauce	500ml	109.5	0.8	1.4	1.00
Asda Garlic & Herb Sauce	275	115.2	0.9	0.9	1.00
Crucials Garlic Flavoured Mayo Dip	500ml	134.7	1.0	1.0	1.00
Crucials Garlic Flavoured Mayo Dip	500ml	134.7	1.0	1.0	1.00
Essential Waitrose Mayonnaise	500ml	190.2	1.3	1.7	1.05
Sainsbury's French Style Mayonnaise	500ml	178.2	1.4	0.9	1.50
Morrisons Mayonnaise	500ml	190.8	1.5	0.6	1.00
Heinz Seriously Good Mayonnaise	680	193.2	1.6	0.9	2.00
Morrisons The Best Mayonnaise	165	206.1	1.6	0.8	1.45
Waitrose Garlic Mayonnaise	250ml	213.3	1.7	2.3	1.71
Sainsbury's Mayonnaise, Thick & Creamy	500ml	219.2	1.7	1.1	0.85
Morrisons Light Mayonnaise	500ml	82.8	1.8	0.6	1.00
Tesco Mayonnaise Real	450ml	223.8	1.8	0.8	0.75
Hellmann's Real Mayonnaise	600	216.3	1.9	0.4	2.00
Sainsbury's Mayonnaise, SO Organic	240ml	225.0	2.7	2.2	1.60
Waitrose Duchy Organic Mayonnaise	250ml	231.9	2.7	1.7	1.75
Asda Real Mayonnaise	500ml	188.4	20.6	0.5	0.70

VALUES SHOWN PER 30 GRAMS SERVING

Sauces (Mustard)

Suggested Brands	Size (g)	Kcal	S.fat (g)	Carbs (g)	£
Skinny Mustard & Honey	425ml	3.6	0.0	0.5	3.99
Essential Waitrose Mustard Piccalilli	460	16.8	0.0	2.7	1.60
Tesco Mustard Piccalilli	350	18.0	0.0	3.9	1.00
Asda Mustard Piccalilli	290	21.9	0.0	4.8	0.79
Asda American Style Mustard	300	13.8	0.1	0.8	1.00
Sainsbury's Honey & Mustard Dressing, Be Good To Yourself	260	23.4	0.1	4.8	0.85
Kamis Spicy Sarepta Mustard	185	27.9	0.1	2.4	0.85
Asda Mild French	185	32.1	0.1	2.3	0.39
Waitrose Mustard With Horseradish	185	34.5	0.1	1.3	1.25
Heinz Yellow Mustard Mild	220	35.4	0.1	2.8	1.69
Heinz Yellow Mild Mustard New York Deli Style	400ml	35.4	0.1	2.8	2.19
Sainsbury's Dark French Mustard	210	36.0	0.1	3.6	0.80
Sainsbury's Horseradish Mustard	205	38.4	0.1	2.5	0.80
Morrisons French Mustard	185	42.3	0.1	3.1	0.65
Maille Wholegrain Mustard	210	52.8	0.1	2.8	1.49

Suggested Brands	Size (g)	Kcal	S.fat (g)	Carbs (g)	£
French's Classic Yellow Mustard	397	21.6	0.2	0.5	1.79
Hellmann's American Style Yellow Mustard	260	34.2	0.2	0.6	2.00
Asda Coarse Grain French Mustard	165	38.7	0.2	1.0	0.34
Essential Waitrose Dijon Mustard	180	42.3	0.2	0.6	0.72
Morrisons The Best Dijon Mustard	190	43.5	0.2	1.2	1.50
Maille Dijon Original Mustard	215	45.0	0.2	1.1	1.49
Tesco American Style Mustard	370	46.5	0.2	6.5	1.40
Morrisons Dijon Mustard	185	47.1	0.2	1.7	0.65
Sainsbury's American Style Mustard	325	48.0	0.2	6.7	1.25
Sainsbury's Dijon Mustard	210	50.4	0.2	1.6	0.80
Heinz English Mustard Classic Style Hot	220ml	50.7	0.2	5.1	1.69
Essential Waitrose Wholegrain Mustard	185	55.5	0.2	1.5	0.75
Morrisons Savers English Mustard	185	56.4	0.2	6.5	0.30
Sainsbury's English Mustard	185	57.3	0.2	5.5	0.65
Sainsbury's English Mustard, Basics	180	57.9	0.2	7.1	0.35
Colman's Original English Mustard	100	58.5	0.2	3.9	1.10

COMMON FOOD SAUCES (MUSTARD)

Suggested Brands	Size (g)	Kcal	S.fat (g)	Carbs (g)	£
Morrisons English Mustard	185	61.5	0.2	6.0	0.60
Sainsbury's Wholegrain Mustard & Chilli	210	65.7	0.2	4.5	0.80
Sainsbury's Wholegrain Mustard & Honey	210	66.0	0.2	5.4	0.80
Morrisons Wholegrain Mustard	175	67.5	0.2	4.5	0.60
Sainsbury's Wholegrain Mustard	205	64.8	0.3	4.2	1.50
Morrisons The Best Whole Grain Mustard	180	43.8	0.4	1.4	1.50
Asda Dijon Mustard	185	46.8	0.4	1.1	0.37
Tesco English Mustard	190	54.9	0.4	4.5	0.55
Tesco Wholegrain Mustard	180	56.4	0.4	2.7	0.55
Tesco Dijon Mustard	185	48.6	0.5	1.4	0.55
Asda Hot English Mustard	180	54.0	0.8	3.6	0.37

VALUES SHOWN PER 30 GRAMS SERVING

Sauces (Peri Peri)

Suggested Brands	Size (g)	Kcal	S.fat (g)	Carbs (g)	£
Nando's Peri-Peri Sauce Medium	250	13.5	0.1	0.3	2.48
Nando's Peri-Peri Sauce Garlic	250	14.7	0.1	12.6	2.48
Sainsbury's Peri Peri Sauce	155	15.6	0.1	1.1	1.00
East End Medium Peri Peri Sauce	250	18.0	0.1	1.9	1.00
East End Garlic Peri Peri Sauce	250	18.3	0.1	2.0	1.00
Nando's Marinade Medium	262	24.6	0.1	2.4	1.99

VALUES SHOWN PER 30 GRAMS SERVING

Sauces (Ranch)

Suggested Brands	Size (g)	Kcal	S.fat (g)	Carbs (g)	£
Sainsbury's Ranch Dressing	250ml	82.8	0.8	3.6	0.85
ASDA Smoky Buttermilk Ranch Dressing	250ml	103.2	0.8	3.2	0.75
Morrisons American Ranch Sauce	330	143.7	1.1	2.9	1.00
Newman's Own Ranch Dressing	250ml	150.0	2.5	2.0	1.60

VALUES SHOWN PER 30 GRAMS SERVING

Sauces (Salad Cream)

Suggested Brands	Size (g)	Kcal	S.fat (g)	Carbs (g)	£
Tesco 50% Less Fat Salad Cream	535	33.9	0.2	4.1	0.90
Stockwell & Co Salad Cream	540	34.5	0.2	4.0	0.61
ASDA Salad Cream 70% Less Fat	420	36.0	0.2	4.2	0.55
ASDA Smart Price Salad Cream	420	36.3	0.2	3.9	0.45
Sainsbury's Salad Cream, Basics	440	41.1	0.2	3.6	0.60
Heinz salad cream 70% reduced fat	435	41.4	0.2	4.6	2.05
Heinz Salad Cream Extra Light	435	41.4	0.2	4.6	2.30
Sainsbury's Salad Cream, Be Good To Yourself	440	54.9	0.3	3.6	0.90
Heinz Salad Cream	605	65.4	0.4	4.6	2.00
Heinz salad cream 30% less fat	415	65.4	0.4	4.6	2.00
Tesco Free From Salad Cream	440	69.6	0.4	5.6	1.00
Morrisons Squeezy Light Salad Cream	450	49.5	0.5	3.1	0.90
Tesco Salad Cream Squeezy	520	66.9	0.5	5.5	0.90
ASDA Free From Salad Cream	295	72.6	0.5	5.1	0.95
essential Waitrose squeezy salad cream	450	85.2	0.5	5.3	1.29

Suggested Brands	Size (g)	Kcal	S.fat (g)	Carbs (g)	£
Heinz Salad Cream Original	605	87.9	0.5	5.6	2.00
ASDA Salad Cream	420	92.7	0.6	5.4	0.55
Sainsbury's Salad Cream	420	99.3	0.6	6.2	0.90

Values Shown Per 30 Grams Serving

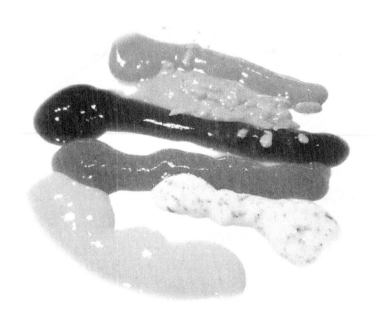

Spices

Suggested Brands	Size (g)	Kcal	S.fat (g)	Carbs (g)	£
Basil	0.7	0	0	0.17	0.01
Rosemary	1.7	1	0	0.7	0.01
Thyme	1.0	3	0	0.4	0.01
Cider Vinegar	14.9	3	0	0.14	0.01
Tarragon	1.8	3	0	2.0	0.01
Red Wine Vinegar	14.9	3	0	4.0	0.01
Black Pepper	2.4	5	0	1.5	0.01
Sage	2	6	0	0.4	0.01
Bay Leaf	8.6	6	0	1.3	0.01
Turmeric	2.2	7	0	1.31	0.01
Balsamic Vinegar	16	14	0	2.72	0.01
Marjoram	1.7	3	0.01	0.33	0.01
Oregano	1	3	0.01	0.44	0.01
Paprika	2.3	6	0.01	0.44	0.01
Anise Seed	2.1	7	0.01	0.75	0.01
Onion Powder	2.4	7	0.01	1.5	0.01
Garlic Powder	3.1	10	0.01	1.95	0.01
Mustard Seed	2	10	0.01	0.35	0.01
Cardamom	5.8	16	0.01	2.37	0.01
Cinnamon	7.9	17	0.01	2.18	0.01
Ground Ginger	5.2	17	0.01	3.02	0.01
Caraway Seeds	6.7	20	0.01	0.83	0.01
Cumin	6	23	0.01	2.04	0.01
Chili Powder	2.7	6	0.1	0.44	0.01
Curry Powder	6.3	20	0.1	0.12	0.01
Nutmeg	2.2	11	0.6	1.95	0.01

AS PER SHOWN SIZE TABLE SPOON GRAM EQUIVALENT

Yogurt Pot

Suggested Brands	Size (g)	Kcal	S.fat (g)	Carbs (g)	£
Onken Light & Fruity Passionfruit	450	76.5	0	9.45	1.40
Total 0% fat free Greek strained	500	81	0	4.5	2.75
Waitrose 1 Greek natural fat free strained	500	97.5	0	8.25	1.89
Fage Total 0% Fat with Peach	170	100.5	0	12.75	1.00
Total 0% fat free Greek yoghurt with strawberry	170	100.5	0	12.6	1.10
Total 0% fat free Greek yoghurt with blueberry	170	100.5	0	12.6	1.10
Yeo Valley Fat Free Greek Style Honey	450	111	0	16.95	1.40
Onken Fat Free Strawberry	450	112.5	0	19.5	1.40
Onken Fat Free Vanilla	450	112.5	0	21	1.40
Onken Fat Free Blueberry & Elderberry	450	118.5	0	21	1.40
Yeo Valley Fat Free Vanilla	450	121.5	0	21.15	1.40
Yeo Valley 0% Fat Vanilla	450	121.5	0	21.15	1.50
Onken Fat Free Apple & Mango	450	123	0	22.5	1.40
Total 0% fat free Greek yoghurt with honey	170	159	0	27	1.10
Liberte Greek Style Blueberry	450	126	0.015	17.7	2.00

Suggested Brands	Size (g)	Kcal	S.fat (g)	Carbs (g)	£
Liberte Greek Style Strawberry	450	126	0.015	18	2.00
Weight Watchers Summer Fruit	440	67.5	0.075	8.85	1.00
Light & Free Fat Free Greek Style Peach Passionfruit	460	67.5	0.075	9.45	1.50
Lancashire Farm Low Fat Natural	1000	72	0.075	10.95	1.50
Light & Free Fat Free Greek Style Lemon	460	73.5	0.075	10.65	1.50
Light & Free Fat Free Greek Style Strawberry	460	75	0.075	10.2	1.50
Light & Free Fat Free Greek Style Cherry	460	76.5	0.075	11.55	1.50
Light & Free Greek Style Fat Free Vanilla Vibe	460	79.5	0.075	10.65	1.50
Light & Free Fat Free Greek Style Raspberry	460	79.5	0.075	11.7	1.50
essential Waitrose fat free Greek style natural	500	81	0.075	7.2	1.05
ASDA Fat Free Rhubarb & Vanilla	450	84	0.075	12	0.92
ASDA Fat Free Cherry	450	84	0.075	12.15	0.92
Arla Skyr Honey	450	105	0.075	10.65	1.40
Liberte Greek Style Strawberry 0% Fat	450	126	0.075	18	2.00
Onken Fat Free Natural Biopot	1000	58.5	0.15	6.3	2.00
Morrisons Fat Free Greek Style	500	70.5	0.15	8.1	0.80

COMMON FOOD   YOGURT POT

Suggested Brands	Size (g)	Kcal	S.fat (g)	Carbs (g)	£
Morrisons Fat Free Natural	500	70.5	0.15	9.6	0.80
essential Waitrose fat free natural	500	75	0.15	9.6	0.95
Muller Light Greek Style Skinny Latte Flavour	450	87	0.15	11.25	1.40
Muller Light Greek Style Luscious Lemon	450	90	0.15	11.25	1.40
Muller Light Greek Style Raspberry	450	90	0.15	11.25	1.40
Muller Light Greek Style Strawberry	450	93	0.15	11.7	1.40
Arla Skyr Strawberry	450	109.5	0.15	11.1	1.40
Sainsbury's Fat Free Natural	500	72	0.3	9.6	0.80
ASDA Fat Free Greek	500	93	0.3	8.25	1.60
Morrisons The Best Greek Yogurt 0% Fat	500	99	0.3	9	1.75
Arla Skyr Vanilla	450	111	0.3	12.45	1.40
Sainsbury's Greek Style Fat Free Natural	500	81	0.45	7.8	0.90
ASDA Greek Style Fat Free	500	82.5	0.45	7.95	0.90
Alpro Natural	500	75	0.6	3.15	1.50
Alpro Soya simply plain plant-based alternative to yogurt	500	75	0.6	3.15	1.50
Alpro Almond	500	81	0.6	3.45	1.50
Light & Free Fat Free Greek Style Coconut	460	82.5	0.6	10.8	1.50

Suggested Brands	Size (g)	Kcal	S.fat (g)	Carbs (g)	£
Muller Light Greek Style Coconut with a Hint of Vanilla	450	94.5	0.6	11.25	1.40
Alpro Yogurt Alternative Cherry	500	112.5	0.6	14.1	1.50
Alpro Vanilla	500	112.5	0.6	14.25	1.50
Lancashire Farm Mango	450	123	0.9	23.25	1.00
Nush Almond Milk Blueberry	120	154.5	0.9	9.9	1.20
ASDA Low Fat Vanilla	450	115.5	1.05	18	0.92
Sainsbury's Low Fat Natural Yogurt, SO Organic	500	88.5	1.2	9.75	1.50
Sainsbury's Low Fat Natural	500	93	1.2	10.65	0.80
essential Waitrose low fat natural	500	91.5	1.35	10.2	0.95
ASDA Low Fat Strawberry	450	124.5	1.35	18	0.89
Activia Low Fat Vanilla Yogurt & Granola	165	168	1.35	27.3	0.75
Activia Low Fat Vanilla Yogurt & Granola	165	168	1.35	27.3	1.00
Benecol Greek Style Big Pot	450	106.5	1.5	6	2.75
Waitrose deliciously nutty hazelnut low fat	150	153	1.5	19.35	0.54
Alpro Coconut	500	82.5	1.65	3.45	1.50
M savers Low Fat Natural	500	87	1.65	8.4	0.45
Sainsbury's Low Fat Natural	500	90	1.65	9.6	0.50

Suggested Brands	Size (g)	Kcal	S.fat (g)	Carbs (g)	£
Total 2% low fat Greek strained	500	105	1.95	4.5	2.75
Waitrose deliciously fruity raspberry low fat	150	133.5	1.95	19.65	0.54
Waitrose deliciously exotic mango & passionfruit low fat	150	142.5	2.1	21.9	0.54
ASDA Strawberry Split	150	133.5	2.4	21	0.35
Morrisons Low Fat Greek Style	500	102	2.55	7.65	0.80
Sainsbury's Greek Style Low Fat Natural	500	112.5	2.55	10.65	0.90
ASDA Cherry Split	150	136.5	2.55	21	0.35
Onken Raspberry	450	142.5	2.55	19.5	1.40
Onken Mango, Papaya & Passion Fruit	450	144	2.55	19.5	1.40
Waitrose deliciously silky toffee low fat	150	145.5	2.55	20.7	0.54
Onken Cherry	450	150	2.55	21	1.40
Onken Strawberry Wholegrain	450	156	2.55	22.5	1.40
Ski Smooth Strawberry & Raspberry	480	124.5	2.7	17.4	1.00
Lancashire Farm Coconut	450	160.5	2.76	26.55	1.00
Morrisons Natural	500	102	2.85	7.65	0.80
essential Waitrose low fat Greek style natural	500	115.5	2.85	10.5	1.05
Glenilen Farm Raspberry	140	118.5	2.85	11.55	0.99
Glenilen Farm Rhubarb	140	118.5	2.85	12.3	0.99
Glenilen Farm Strawberry	140	121.5	2.85	12.6	0.99

Suggested Brands	Size (g)	Kcal	S.fat (g)	Carbs (g)	£
Glenilen Farm Mango & Passionfruit	140	123	2.85	12.75	0.99
Sainsbury's Fab Creamy Hazelnut	150	189	3	21.45	0.50
ASDA Berry Granola Split	135	190.5	3	27	0.35
Morrisons Mango, Papaya & Passion Fruit Bio	450	156	3.45	22.35	0.85
Rumi Turkish Yogurt	1000	78	3.6	6.45	1.15
Yeo Valley Lemon Curd	450	172.5	3.75	23.4	1.40
Yeo Valley Organic Whole Milk Lemon Curd	450	172.5	3.75	23.4	1.50
Yeo Valley Banana & Custard	450	142.5	3.9	15.6	1.40
Yeo Valley Strawberry	450	147	4.2	16.35	1.40
Yeo Valley Raspberry	450	148.5	4.2	16.65	1.50
The Collective Super Berries	450	177	4.95	20.4	2.20
The Collective Passion Fruit	450	180	5.1	19.35	2.20
The Collective Raspberry	450	180	5.1	21	2.20
ASDA Banana Flakes Split	135	213	5.1	28.5	0.35
Rachel's organic forbidden fruits peach	150	174	5.25	19.05	0.75
Rachel's organic forbidden fruits cherry	150	175.5	5.25	19.5	0.75
ASDA Chocolate Balls Split	135	207	5.25	27	0.35
Fage Total Greek Natural	500	139.5	5.4	4.5	2.75
Total Greek strained natural	500	139.5	5.4	4.5	2.75

COMMON FOOD   YOGURT POT

Suggested Brands	Size (g)	Kcal	S.fat (g)	Carbs (g)	£
The Collective Dairy Cherry	450	180	5.4	19.95	2.20
The Collective Banana & Butterscotch	450	198	5.4	22.95	2.20
ASDA Toffee Hoops Split	135	229.5	5.55	31.5	0.35
Waitrose Duchy Organic thick & creamy natural	500	150	5.7	9.9	1.57
Sainsbury's West Country Black Cherry Yogurt	150	186	5.85	20.55	0.70
Waitrose black cherry	150	187.5	6	20.4	0.80
Waitrose Mango & Papaya	150	178.5	6.15	18.3	0.80
Waitrose Mango & Papaya	150	178.5	6.15	18.3	0.80
Waitrose Scottish raspberry	150	187.5	6.15	19.35	0.80
Sainsbury's West Country Timperley Rhubarb	150	169.5	6.3	15.15	0.70
Sainsbury's West Country Mango & Yuzu Yogurt	150	207	6.45	24.15	0.70
Sainsbury's West Country Senga Strawberry	150	177	6.6	16.05	0.70
Sainsbury's Pink Grapefruit & Gin West Country	150	180	6.75	18.15	0.75
Rachel's organic Greek style ginger	450	196.5	6.75	19.65	2.10
Waitrose Madagascan vanilla	150	187.5	6.9	17.7	0.80
Rachel's organic Greek style honey	450	196.5	6.9	19.05	2.10

Suggested Brands	Size (g)	Kcal	S.fat (g)	Carbs (g)	£
Waitrose honey & stem ginger	150	198	6.9	20.25	0.80
Sainsbury's West Country Glen Ample Raspberry	150	187.5	7.05	16.8	0.70
Tesco Greek Style Vanilla Yogurt	450	187.5	7.2	19.05	1.00
Sainsbury's West Country Spanish Honey & Ginger	150	207	7.2	21.6	0.70
Yeo Valley Greek Style Honey	450	211.5	7.2	20.55	1.40
Sainsbury's West Country Creamy Fudge Yogurt	150	217.5	7.2	24.9	0.70
Sainsbury's Pineapple & Coconut	150	183	7.35	18.3	0.70
St Helen's Farm natural goats milk	450	157.5	7.5	6.45	2.40
Sainsbury's West Country Madagascan Vanilla	150	198	7.5	17.85	0.70
Waitrose Sea Salt Caramel	150	214.5	7.5	23.1	0.80
Sainsbury's Hazelnut	150	243	7.5	22.5	0.70
Oykos Apple & Cinnamon Greek Style	440	210	7.65	20.25	2.00
Tesco Greek Style Honey	450	216	7.8	20.55	1.00
Tesco Greek Style Coconut	450	184.5	7.95	15.15	1.00
Rachel's organic Greek style coconut	450	201	7.95	16.05	2.10
Oykos Peach Greek Style	440	204	7.95	19.2	2.00
Oykos Raspberry Greek Style	440	213	7.95	20.85	2.00

Suggested Brands	Size (g)	Kcal	S.fat (g)	Carbs (g)	£
Oykos Strawberry Greek Style	440	217.5	7.95	22.2	2.00
Oykos Tiramisu Greek Style	440	241.5	7.95	27	2.00
Waitrose lemon curd	150	235.5	8.1	24.75	0.80
Sainsbury's West Country Lemon Curd Yogurt	150	249	8.1	28.65	0.70
Morrisons Greek Style Honey	200	213	8.25	20.4	0.55
Tims Dairy Greek style yogurt with honey	175	226.5	8.25	21.3	0.61
Rachel's organic Greek style natural set	450	174	8.4	7.5	2.10
Oykos Salted Caramel Greek Style	440	229.5	8.4	24.3	2.00
Tims Dairy Greek style yogurt with vanilla	450	229.5	8.7	19.35	1.30
essential Waitrose Greek style natural	500	183	9.15	8.1	1.05
Tims Dairy Greek style natural	500	195	9.6	7.35	1.23
ASDA Greek Style	500	187.5	10.05	7.35	0.90
Waitrose 1 Greek natural strained	500	196.5	10.05	5.55	1.89
Morrisons The Best Greek Yogurt 10% Fat	500	196.5	10.65	6.45	1.75
Morrisons Greek Style Yogurt	500	189	10.95	6	0.80
ASDA Authentic Greek	500	195	11.4	5.7	1.60
Fage Total Fat Free Greek Recipe Natural	500	81	13.5	4.5	2.75

COMMON FOOD

Suggested Brands	Size (g)	Kcal	S.fat (g)	Carbs (g)	£
Co Yo Natural Coconut Milk Yoghurt	400	352.5	30	5.85	3.99

Values Shown Per 150 Gram Serving

Find Us On

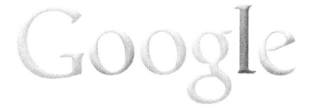

Search: **NADIET.INFO**

Notes

Fish

If you have cholesterol issues and taking statin medication, your doctor will have recommended avoidance of shellfish including shrimp, crayfish, crab, lobster, clams, scallops, oysters, and mussels. All these foods are high in vitamin B12 and dietary cholesterol.

Avoiding shellfish over a long time can result in a lack of B12 in the blood stream. This results in your doctor either prescribing medication in daily tablet form, or having a monthly B12 injection provided by a registered nurse. When taking prescribed statin type medication over a long period of time, the body will stop absorbing vitamin B12 irritating the vitamin deficiency.

My view is to try different types of fish and find your favourite, if this is shellfish, eat small amounts and enjoy the meal. This is a much better solution than avoiding shellfish completely and risking vitamin B12 deficiency. Research is starting to prove that high levels of dietary cholesterol in shellfish, milk, eggs and liver are good for HDL (good) cholesterol rather than encouraging LDL (bad) cholesterol to increase.

I believe by 2025 foods containing high dietary cholesterol will be encouraged in our daily diets, compared to the 1990's when we were taught to avoid high dietary cholesterol foods that would result in heart issues.

Cod (Battered)

Suggested Brands	Size (g)	Kcal	S.fat (g)	Carbs (g)	£
Birds Eye 4 Large Battered Cod Fillets	440	253.0	0.6	18.7	4.80
Morrisons 4 Battered Chunky Cod Fillet	500	220.0	0.8	19.1	3.60
Sainsbury's 4 Chunky Battered Cod	500	241.3	0.8	20.0	3.00
Arctic Royal 2 Jumbo Battered Cod Fillets	500	417.5	0.8	38.5	6.00
Iceland Battered 4 Chunky Cod Fillets	500	202.5	1.0	15.6	3.00
Tesco Plant 2 Chef Battered Fish Free Fillets	250	291.3	1.0	30.9	3.00
Iceland 4 Battered Whitefish Fillets	400	196.0	1.1	19.3	1.75
Iceland 6 Battered Cod Fillets	750	233.8	1.1	22.5	4.00
Tesco 4 Battered Chunky Cod Fillets	500	257.5	1.1	17.3	3.25
Morrisons 6 Large Battered Cod Fillets	750	265.0	1.1	21.8	3.50
Waitrose Frozen 2 battered cod fillets	300	268.5	1.2	21.9	3.40
Young's 2 Tempura Crispy & Golden Battered Cod Fillets	300	270.0	1.2	17.7	2.50
Tesco Finest 2 Beer Battered Cod Fillets	385	239.7	1.3	16.9	4.50
Birds Eye 4 Battered Fish Fillets	400	244.0	1.3	17.0	2.85

Fish   Cod (Battered)

Suggested Brands	Size (g)	Kcal	S.fat (g)	Carbs (g)	£
Tesco 4 Battered Cod Fillets	500	292.5	1.3	20.5	3.00
Sainsbury's 4 Battered Cod	500	316.3	1.3	24.1	2.65
Young's Gastro Tempura Battered 2 Lemon & Herb Basa Fillets	310	252.7	1.4	14.6	4.00
Birds Eye 2 Cod Fillets in Original Batter	284	295.4	1.6	22.7	4.50
Birds Eye Inspirations 2 Chunky Cod Fillets in a Signature Golden Batter	284	295.4	1.6	22.7	4.50
Morrisons 2 Market St Battered Cod Fillets	300	343.5	2.0	31.8	3.50
Waitrose 2 Bubbly Battered Cod	380	416.1	2.1	25.7	4.99
Tesco 2 Extra Large Battered Cod Fillets	400	522.0	2.4	40.6	3.25
Young's Chip Shop 4 Large Cod Fillets	440	271.7	2.8	16.2	3.00

Values shown per fillet

Cod (Breaded)

Suggested Brands	Size (g)	Kcal	S.fat (g)	Carbs (g)	£
Sainsbury's Breaded Chunky Cod Fillets, Be Good To Yourself x4	500	195.0	0.3	20.5	3.00
Morrisons 4 Chunky Breaded Cod Fillets	500	208.8	0.6	18.0	3.60
Birds Eye 4 Breaded Cod Large Fillets	440	232.1	0.7	24.2	3.75
Tesco 2 Breaded Chunky Cod Fillets	350	278.3	0.7	22.2	3.20
Morrisons The Best Chunky Breaded Cod Fillets x 2	350	329.0	0.7	29.9	3.50
ASDA 4 Breaded Cod Fillets	500	225.0	0.8	21.3	2.98
Tesco 4 Breaded Chunky Prime Cod Fillets	500	245.0	0.8	22.1	3.25
Waitrose 4 MSC line caught prime cod fillet in breadcrumbs	500	247.5	0.8	20.1	7.49
ASDA 2 Crisp Crumb Chunky Cod Fillets	350	276.5	0.9	17.5	3.20
Tesco 4 Breaded Cod Fillets	500	278.8	0.9	27.4	2.75
Iceland 6 Breaded Cod Fillets	750	221.3	1.0	20.8	4.00
Waitrose Frozen 2 breaded cod fillets	300	273.0	1.1	22.1	3.25
Sainsbury's Breaded Cod Fillets x2	300	286.5	1.1	27.5	3.00

FISH   COD (BREADED)

Suggested Brands	Size (g)	Kcal	S.fat (g)	Carbs (g)	£
Morrisons Market St Breaded Cod Fillets x 2	285	306.4	1.1	26.4	2.50
ASDA 2 Crisp Crumb Cod Fillets	284	308.1	1.1	29.8	1.98
Young's Lightly Breaded 2 Chunky Cod Fillets	250	225.0	1.3	17.8	2.50
Young's 4 Large Breaded Cod Fillets	480	261.6	2.2	22.6	3.50
Youngs Simply Breaded 4 Large Cod Fillets	440	255.2	2.5	15.4	4.50

VALUES SHOWN PER FILLET

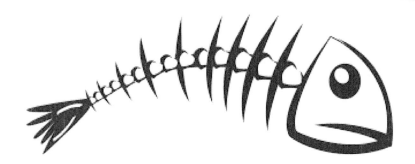

Cod (Fillet)

Suggested Brands	Size (g)	Kcal	S.fat (g)	Carbs (g)	£
ASDA Line Caught 2 Cod Fillets	260	130.0	0.0	1.3	3.19
Tesco Cod Fillets x 4	360	72.0	0.1	0.0	3.70
Waitrose MSC Icelandic cod fillet x 4	500	90.0	0.1	0.1	7.99
4 x Fresh Skinless & Boneless British Cod Fillets	500	92.5	0.1	0.0	10.99
Waitrose 2 MSC skinless, boneless cod fillets	240	122.4	0.1	1.2	4.99
Morrisons Market St 2 Cod Fillets	250	122.5	0.1	0.6	4.00
Waitrose Frozen 2 British Cod Fillet Portions MSC	280	126.0	0.1	0.0	6.00
Waitrose Frozen 4 MSC line caught cod fillets	475	127.1	0.1	1.2	5.99
ASDA Extra Special Cod Loin	260	200.2	0.1	2.6	4.00
ASDA 4 Cod Fillets	400	75.0	0.2	0.0	3.00
Iceland 4 Atlantic Cod Fillets	450	84.4	0.2	0.0	4.50
Tesco 2 Boneless Cod Fillets	280	112.0	0.3	0.0	3.95
Young's Skinless & Boneless Atlantic Cod Chunky Fillets x4	360	88.2	0.4	0.0	4.25
Sainsbury's Cod Fillets, Boneless & Skinless	250	122.5	0.4	0.0	3.40

Values Shown Per Fillet

Crab

Suggested Brands	Size (g)	Kcal	S.fat (g)	Carbs (g)	£
Ocean Isle Premium Crab Meat	100	77.1	0.1	0.2	4.00
Ocean Finest Crab Claw Meat	114	87.9	0.1	0.2	4.00
Kingfisher Whole Lump Crab Meat	105	84.0	0.2	1.6	2.80
Kingfisher Catch Shredded Crab Meat	145	65.3	0.3	1.2	2.00
Kingfisher Jumbo Crab	145	116.0	0.3	2.2	2.85
John West Crab Meat Chunks	170	119.0	0.3	2.2	3.50
Orkney Crab Meat	100	108.0	1.3	1.1	3.50
ASDA 16 Seafood Sticks	250	297.5	1.3	45.0	0.84

VALUES SHOWN PER PRODUCT

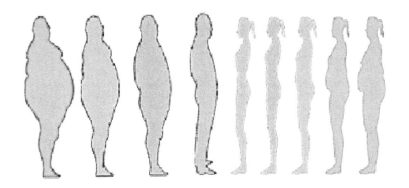

Fish Cakes

Suggested Brands	Size (g)	Kcal	S.fat (g)	Carbs (g)	£
Young's Gastro 8 Mini Fishcakes Spicy Salmon & Black Bean with a Chipotle Chilli Salsa Dip	280	69.3	0.3	6.4	3.50
Birds Eye 4 Breaded Cod Cakes	198	90.1	0.3	7.4	1.10
Birds Eye Cod Fish Cakes 4 Pack	198	90.1	0.3	7.4	1.10
Waitrose Prawn & Sweet Potato Fishcakes x 2	290	197.2	0.3	24.9	2.99
Youngs Flipper Dippers 10 Pack	250	52.0	0.4	6.1	1.49
Iceland 10 Breaded Cod Fishcakes	420	100.0	0.4	9.7	1.00
Slimming World Free Food 2 Thai Style Fishcakes	280	119.0	0.4	7.3	2.50
Hearty Food Co Pollock Fishcakes X 4	340	128.4	0.4	15.6	1.80
Tesco 2 Smoked Haddock Fishcakes	270	207.9	0.5	24.2	1.75
Tesco 2 Cod Fishcake With Lemon&Herb	270	213.3	0.5	25.2	1.75
Hearty Food Co 10 Cod Fishcakes	500	90.5	0.6	10.2	1.25
ASDA 4 Quarter Pounder Salmon Burgers	456	197.2	0.6	22.8	3.00
Tesco Finest 2 Thai Prawn Fishcakes	290	210.3	0.6	21.2	2.65

FISH   FISH CAKES

Suggested Brands	Size (g)	Kcal	S.fat (g)	Carbs (g)	£
Tesco Finest 2 Cod Sweet Potato And Chilli Fishcakes	290	216.1	0.6	24.8	2.65
ASDA 8 Breaded Cod Fishcakes	400	88.5	0.7	9.0	1.80
Morrisons 8 Cod Fish Cakes	400	92.5	0.7	9.9	1.20
Birds Eye 2 Cod Fish Fillet Burgers	227	231.5	0.7	23.8	2.00
Tesco Meat Free 4 Fishless Fishcakes	360	241.2	0.7	33.0	1.75
Morrisons Fishmonger Smoked Haddock Fishcakes 2	270	247.1	0.7	23.9	1.30
Gastro 8 Mini Fishcakes Smoked Haddock Arancini Style	280	79.1	0.8	6.4	3.50
Young's Omega 3 12 Fish Cakes	600	96.0	0.8	9.5	2.00
Sainsbury's Cod Fishcakes x2	170	164.9	0.8	14.9	1.25
Morrisons 2 Cod Fish Cakes	270	248.4	0.8	25.4	1.30
Sainsbury's Mediterranean Tuna Fishcakes, Taste the Difference X 2	300	259.5	0.8	27.2	2.50
ASDA 8 Battered Cod Fishcakes	360	102.6	0.9	8.1	1.80
ASDA 4 Cod Fishcakes	460	186.3	0.9	20.7	2.70

Suggested Brands	Size (g)	Kcal	S.fat (g)	Carbs (g)	£
ASDA Extra Special 2 Cod & Prawn Red Thai Fishcakes	290	234.9	1.0	26.1	1.97
Sainsbury's Pacific Salmon Fishcakes x2	170	179.4	1.1	15.0	1.25
Waitrose Vegan Fish'less'cakes X 2	235	188.0	1.1	20.3	2.99
Morrisons Market St Gluten Free Cod Fishcakes X 2	270	260.6	1.1	27.1	1.30
essential Waitrose MSC cod & parsley fish cakes	170	164.9	1.2	13.0	1.40
Tesco Free From Cod And Parsley Fishcake X 2	270	220.1	1.2	26.3	1.75
Waitrose Gluten Free Cod Fishcakes x 2	290	237.8	1.2	29.9	2.99
Waitrose Frozen 2 Thai prawn fish cakes	230	200.1	1.3	21.6	2.99
ASDA 4 Salmon Fishcakes	460	208.2	1.3	19.6	2.70
Morrisons 2 Cod & Chive Fish Cakes	230	197.8	1.4	23.0	1.75
Waitrose Frozen salmon & dill fish cakes x 2	230	222.0	1.4	16.0	2.99
Sainsbury's Fishcakes Haddock x2	270	249.8	1.4	23.2	1.45
ASDA 4 Smoked Haddock Fishcakes	460	201.3	1.5	20.7	2.70
Waitrose MSC frozen smoked haddock fish cakes x 2	230	238.1	1.5	18.5	2.99

FISH   FISH CAKES

Suggested Brands	Size (g)	Kcal	S.fat (g)	Carbs (g)	£
ASDA 2 Crisp Crumb Smoked Haddock Fishcakes	270	243.0	1.5	25.7	1.39
Sainsbury's Deliciously Free From Haddock Fishcakes X 2	270	243.0	1.5	21.3	2.40
ASDA 2 Crisp Crumb Cod & Parsley Fishcakes	270	253.8	1.5	24.3	1.39
ASDA 4 Crisp Crumb Cod Fishcakes	540	253.8	1.5	24.3	2.70
ASDA 2 Crisp Crumb Salmon Fishcakes	270	272.7	1.5	24.3	1.39
Morrisons The Best Chunky Thai Salmon & Prawn Fishcakes x 2	290	295.8	1.5	30.2	2.60
Morrisons Fishmonger Salmon Fishcakes 2	270	299.7	1.6	27.1	1.30
Morrisons The Best Salmon & Cod Fishcake With Sweet Chilli Sauce x 2	290	335.0	1.6	41.5	2.60
Sainsbury's Fishcakes Salmon & Ginger, Taste the Difference x2	300	312.0	1.7	26.7	2.50
ASDA Free From 2 Salmon & Dill Fishcakes	180	217.8	1.8	16.2	2.20
Waitrose Easy To Cook 2 Scottish salmon fishcakes with sweet chilli sauce	270	237.6	1.8	23.1	4.19

FISH FISH CAKES

Suggested Brands	Size (g)	Kcal	S.fat (g)	Carbs (g)	£
Sainsbury's Deliciously Free From Thai-Style Haddock Fishcakes x2	170	206.6	1.9	19.7	2.00
Tesco Finest 2 Cod And Parsley Fishcakes	290	246.5	2.0	27.3	2.00
Waitrose Easy to Cook 2 cod fish cakes with cheddar & lemon	315	261.5	2.0	25.5	4.19
Sainsbury's Thai Salmon Fishcakes Sweet Chilli Glaze X 2	307	333.1	2.1	23.5	3.25
The Saucy Fish Co. Smoked Haddock Fishcakes x2	270	220.1	2.2	24.3	2.25
essential Waitrose Cod Fishcakes x 2	270	228.2	2.2	23.1	1.75
essential Waitrose Smoked Haddock Fishcakes x 2	270	253.8	2.2	28.9	1.75
Sainsbury's Cod Fishcakes x2	270	243.0	2.3	20.8	1.45
Sainsbury's Fishcakes King Prawn & Lemongrass, Taste the Difference x2	300	265.5	2.3	30.8	2.25
Morrisons Mediterranean Fish Burgers x 2	188	165.4	2.4	2.8	4.00
The Saucy Fish Co. Salmon & Cod Fishcakes x2	270	267.3	2.4	24.3	2.25
Sainsbury's Fishcakes Scottish Salmon x2	270	286.2	2.4	23.0	1.45

FISH   FISH CAKES

Suggested Brands	Size (g)	Kcal	S.fat (g)	Carbs (g)	£
ASDA Extra Special 2 Melt-in-the-Middle Cod Fishcakes with Tartare Sauce	290	245.1	2.5	24.7	2.50
Tesco Finest 2 Beer Battered Cod Fillets	385	479.3	2.5	33.9	4.50
Tesco Finest 2 Salmon Spinach And Lemon Fishcakes	290	323.4	2.6	25.5	2.00
Iceland Luxury Melt in the Middle Cod Mornay Fish Cakes x 2	260	253.5	2.7	27.4	2.00
ASDA Extra Special 2 Melt-in-the-Middle Salmon Fishcakes with Thai Sauce	290	271.2	2.8	24.7	2.50
Sainsbury's Deliciously Free From Pacific Salmon Fishcakes X 2	270	284.9	2.8	20.9	2.40
Tesco Finest 2 Cod And Chorizo Fishcakes	290	246.5	2.9	20.0	2.65
Sainsbury's Deliciously Free From Cod & Parsley Melting Middle Fishcakes X 2	280	249.2	2.9	19.2	2.75
Morrisons The Best Saucy Smoked Haddock & Davidstow Cheddar Fishcakes x 2	290	268.3	3.0	23.3	2.60
Morrisons The Best 2 Cod & Parsley Sauce Fish Cakes	290	268.3	3.0	23.3	2.60

Suggested Brands	Size (g)	Kcal	S.fat (g)	Carbs (g)	£
Waitrose Smoked Haddock, Cheddar Fishcakes x 2	290	272.6	3.0	26.7	2.99
Morrisons The Best Naked Smoked Haddock & Applewood Cheddar Fishcakes 2	290	224.8	3.2	16.5	2.60
ASDA Extra Special 2 Smoked Haddock Fishcakes with Vintage Cheddar & Leek	290	277.0	3.2	21.8	1.97
Sainsbury's Fishcakes Melting Middle Cod & Parsley Sauce Fishcakes Taste the Difference x2	290	287.1	3.2	26.8	2.50
Sainsbury's Taste the Difference 4 Cod & Parsley Melting Middle Fishcakes	580	287.1	3.2	26.8	3.50
Morrisons 2 Salmon & Broccoli Fish Cakes	460	469.2	3.2	43.7	1.75
Waitrose Salmon, Rocket & Watercress Fishcakes x 2	290	310.3	3.3	27.6	2.99
Iceland Luxury Melt In Middle 2 Smoked Haddock Fish Cakes With A Cheddar With A cheddar Cheese & Parsley Sauce	260	241.8	3.4	21.7	2.00
Morrisons The Best Salmon,Smoked Cod &	290	242.2	3.5	18.3	2.60

FISH   FISH CAKES

Suggested Brands	Size (g)	Kcal	S.fat (g)	Carbs (g)	£
Haddock Fishcakes With Cheddar Sauce X2					
Gastro 2 Melting Middle Chunky Cod with A Creamy Rocket Mornay Sauce Fish Cakes	270	251.1	3.5	21.5	2.50
Waitrose Cod & Parsley Sauce Fishcakes x 2	290	265.4	3.5	24.5	2.99
Morrisons The Best Cod & Chorizo Chunky Fishcake x 2	290	281.3	3.5	24.7	2.60
ASDA Extra Special 2 Cod & Spanish Chorizo Fishcakes	290	290.0	3.5	21.8	1.97
Waitrose Frozen salmon & watercress fish cakes 2s	290	274.1	3.6	23.2	3.69
Waitrose Frozen 2 cod Mornay fish cakes	290	262.5	3.8	22.5	3.69
Tesco Finest 2 Smoked Haddock Fishcakes	290	262.5	3.9	25.5	2.65
Sainsbury's Fishcakes Melting Middle Smoked Haddock with Cheddar & Leek Taste the Difference x2	290	290.0	3.9	25.8	2.00
Sainsbury's Taste the Difference 4 Melting Middle Smoked Haddock Fishcakes	580	290.0	3.9	25.8	3.50

Suggested Brands	Size (g)	Kcal	S.fat (g)	Carbs (g)	£
Morrisons The Best Chunky Salmon and Spinach Fishcakes x 2	290	362.5	3.9	24.5	2.60
Gastro Melting Middle 2 Chunky Smoked Haddock Fish Cakes	270	263.3	4.1	19.2	2.50
ASDA Extra Special 2 Melt-in-the-Middle Smoked Haddock Fishcakes with Rarebit	290	263.9	4.1	23.2	2.50
ASDA Extra Special 2 Smoked Haddock Fishcakes with Cheddar & Mustard	290	310.3	5.1	26.1	1.97
ASDA Extra Special Melting Layer 2 Salmon Fishcakes with Hollandaise Sauce	290	308.9	5.4	24.7	1.97

VALUES SHOWN PER FISH CAKE

Fish Fingers

Suggested Brands	Size (g)	Kcal	S.fat (g)	Carbs (g)	£
Quorn 10 Meat Free Vegan Fishless Fingers	200	42.8	0.1	5.8	2.50
Iceland No Fish Fingers 6 Crispy Coated Fingers	180	51.0	0.1	5.4	2.00
30 Breaded Fish Fingers	750	48.5	0.2	4.5	2.00
Hearty Food Co 10 Fish Fingers	250	57.8	0.2	4.5	0.69
Birds Eye Gluten Free Fish Fingers x12	360	60.9	0.2	5.1	3.00
Birds Eye 10 Omega 3 Fish Fingers	280	61.0	0.2	5.9	2.00
Birds Eye 10 Fish Fingers Cod	280	61.3	0.2	5.9	3.00
Birds Eye 10 Fish Fingers Haddock	280	62.7	0.2	6.2	2.75
Tesco Free From 10 Crispy Cod Fish Fingers	300	63.6	0.2	5.0	2.50
Sainsbury's Deliciously Free From Cod Fish Fingers X 10	300	64.2	0.2	4.8	2.50
Tesco Cod Fish Fingers 10 Pack	300	69.6	0.2	5.3	1.75
ASDA Smart Price 10 Fish Fingers	250	50.5	0.3	4.8	0.69
Sainsbury's Fish Fingers, Basics x10	250	51.5	0.3	4.5	0.80
Sainsbury's 10 Breaded Omega 3 Pollock Fillet Fish Fingers	300	56.1	0.3	4.8	1.00

Suggested Brands	Size (g)	Kcal	S.fat (g)	Carbs (g)	£
Tesco Omega Fish Fingers 10 Pack	300	56.4	0.3	4.8	1.20
Sainsbury's Cod Fish Fingers x12	360	56.4	0.3	4.8	2.00
Morrisons 20 Breaded Cod Fish Fingers	600	59.4	0.3	5.2	3.20
essential Waitrose MSC cod fillet fish fingers x 10	300	60.0	0.3	5.6	1.75
Young's 10 Omega 3 Free From Fish Fingers	300	60.0	0.3	5.2	2.18
ASDA 10 Omega 3 Fish Fingers	300	60.9	0.3	5.7	1.36
Birds Eye 8 Crispy Battered Fish Fingers	224	70.3	0.3	5.6	1.00
Young's Gastro 8 Panko Breaded Chunky Cod Fish Fingers	320	78.0	0.3	6.2	3.00
Youngs Gastro 8 Chunky Breaded Haddock Fingers	320	79.2	0.3	6.3	2.50
Young's Gastro 8 Tempura Battered Chunky	320	80.0	0.4	5.5	3.00
Waitrose Frozen 6 chunky breaded haddock fingers	300	107.0	0.4	10.3	3.25
Sainsbury's Cod Fillet Fish Fingers x6	300	109.0	0.4	9.5	2.95
Sainsbury's Chunky Cod Fish Fingers, Taste the Difference x8	480	120.0	0.4	9.1	3.50
Birds Eye 6 Chunky Fish Fingers Extra Large	360	123.6	0.4	12.0	3.00

FISH   FISH FINGERS

Suggested Brands	Size (g)	Kcal	S.fat (g)	Carbs (g)	£
Sainsbury's Taste the Difference 8 Chunky Haddock Fillet Fish Fingers X 8	480	129.6	0.4	11.6	3.25
Morrisons Free From 10 Cod Fish Fingers	300	64.2	0.5	3.8	2.50
Waitrose Frozen 6 chunky battered haddock fingers	300	112.0	0.5	8.5	3.25
Waitrose Frozen 6 chunky breaded cod fingers	400	142.0	0.5	14.0	3.25
Tesco Finest 6 Chunky Cod Fillet Fish Fingers	400	147.3	0.5	11.5	3.00
Waitrose 6 Chunky Cod Fish Fingers	330	116.1	0.6	11.6	4.50

VALUES SHOWN PER FISH FINGER

Haddock (Battered)

Suggested Brands	Size (g)	Kcal	S.fat (g)	Carbs (g)	£
ASDA 4 Battered Haddock Fillets	500	207.5	0.6	18.8	3.20
Iceland Battered 6 Haddock Skinless Boneless Fillets	750	238.8	1.0	22.1	4.00
Sainsbury's 4 Chunky Battered Haddock	500	276.3	1.1	17.4	3.00
Birds Eye 4 Battered Haddock Fillets	440	257.4	1.3	18.7	4.80
Waitrose Frozen 2 battered haddock fillets	300	285.0	1.4	22.1	3.40
Tesco 4 Battered Haddock Fillets	500	311.3	1.4	20.3	3.00
Waitrose 2 Bubbly Beer Battered Scottish Haddock	380	418.0	2.3	25.7	4.99
essential Waitrose 2 Battered Haddock	250	227.5	2.4	13.9	3.50
Young's 2 Chip Shop Haddock Fillets in Our Crisp Bubbly Batter	220	247.5	2.6	16.3	2.00
Young's Chip Shop 4 Large Haddock Fillets	440	247.5	2.6	16.3	3.00
Young's Chip Shop 2 Extra Large Battered Haddock Fillets	320	350.4	3.2	26.4	4.00

VALUES SHOWN PER FILLET

Haddock (Breaded)

Suggested Brands	Size (g)	Kcal	S.fat (g)	Carbs (g)	£
ASDA 4 Breaded Haddock Fillets	500	216.3	0.6	22.5	3.20
Birds Eye 4 Breaded Haddock Large Fillets	440	236.5	0.7	24.2	3.75
Morrisons 4 Chunky Breaded Haddock Fillets	500	218.8	0.8	16.0	3.60
Waitrose Frozen 2 breaded haddock fillets	300	262.5	0.8	21.5	3.25
Morrisons The Best 2 Chunky Breaded Haddock Fillets	325	297.4	0.8	26.7	3.50
Tesco 2 Breaded Chunky Haddock Fillets	350	334.3	0.9	27.7	3.20
Waitrose MSC line caught prime haddock fillet in breadcrumbs x 4	500	228.8	1.0	15.5	7.74
Tesco 4 Breaded Haddock Fillets	500	307.5	1.0	31.1	2.75
ASDA 2 Crisp Crumb Haddock Fillets	284	301.0	1.1	28.4	1.98
Tesco 4 Breaded Chunky Prime Haddock Fillets	500	253.8	1.6	24.5	3.25
Young's 4 Large Breaded Haddock Fillets	480	244.8	1.9	21.1	3.50
Young's Chip Shop 4 Large Battered Haddock Fillets	480	262.8	2.5	17.6	4.00

VALUES SHOWN PER FILLET

Haddock (Fillets)

Suggested Brands	Size (g)	Kcal	S.fat (g)	Carbs (g)	£
Morrisons 4 Haddock Fillets	360	61.2	0.1	0.0	3.50
Iceland 4 Smoked Haddock Fillets (4)	460	71.3	0.1	0.0	4.50
Iceland 4 Haddock Fillets	400	75.0	0.1	0.0	4.50
Waitrose Fresh Boneless Haddock Fillets (1)	105	84.0	0.1	0.0	1.82
Sainsbury's Smoked Haddock Fillets (4)	400	86.0	0.1	0.0	4.50
Tesco Boneless Haddock Fillets (2)	280	112.0	0.1	0.0	3.95
Waitrose Frozen MSC line caught haddock fillets (4)	425	113.7	0.1	1.1	5.99
Morrisons Market St 2 Haddock Fillets	230	113.9	0.1	0.6	4.00
ASDA 2 Haddock Fillets	240	115.2	0.1	1.2	3.95
ASDA 2 Smoked Haddock Fillets	220	134.2	0.1	1.1	3.19
Waitrose Smoked Haddock Fillets MSC (2)	240	92.4	0.2	1.2	4.99
Sainsbury's Haddock Fillet Portion (4)	380	99.8	0.2	0.0	3.75
Sainsbury's Skinless & Boneless Smoked Haddock Fillets (2)	240	117.6	0.2	0.0	4.50
Tesco 4 Smoked Haddock Fillets	360	52.2	0.3	0.0	3.30
Counter Haddock Fillet tesco	140	102.2	0.3	0.0	1.75

FISH   HADDOCK (FILLETS)

Suggested Brands	Size (g)	Kcal	S.fat (g)	Carbs (g)	£
Tesco 5 Haddock Fillets	400	69.6	0.4	0.3	3.30
Sainsbury's Skinless & Boneless Haddock Fillets (2)	260	150.8	0.4	0.0	4.25
ASDA Smoked Haddock Fillet (1)	105	117.6	1.2	1.1	1.95

VALUES SHOWN PER FILLET

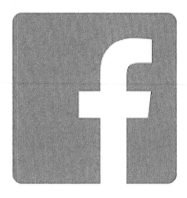

www.facebook.com/StephenddDBarnes

Salmon (Fillets)

Suggested Brands	Size (g)	Kcal	S.fat (g)	Carbs (g)	£
Tesco 5 Wild Alaskan Salmon	550	126	0.8	0.3	5.00
Young's 4 Pacific Pink Salmon Fillets	360	143	0.9	0.0	4.30
Iceland 2 Lemon & Pepper Salmon Portions	250	179	1.0	2.7	2.50
ASDA 2 Wild Keta Salmon Fillets	230	164	1.2	0.1	3.95
ASDA Cook from Frozen Salmon Fillets	360	131	1.4	0.1	3.00
ASDA Smoked Salmon	120	163	1.5	0.6	3.00
Tesco 2 Boneless Salmon Fillets	260	209	1.6	1.6	3.60
Counter Salmon Fillet	240	222	2.0	0.0	3.36
Iceland 4 Wild Pink Salmon Fillets	480	179	2.1	0.0	4.00
Iceland Luxury 2 Lightly Smoked Salmon Fillets	240	203	2.1	1.8	4.50
ASDA 2 Salmon Fillets	240	225	2.1	0.1	3.30
ASDA 2 Lemon & Parsley Steamed Salmon	180	234	2.1	0.1	3.99
ASDA Smoked Salmon Trimmings	120	198	2.2	0.1	1.65
ASDA 2 Salmon Fillets in a Sweet Chilli Dressing	290	203	2.2	6.5	4.50
Iceland Fish Market Salmon x 4	520	217	2.8	0.0	8.00

Fish Salmon (Fillets)

Suggested Brands	Size (g)	Kcal	S.fat (g)	Carbs (g)	£
Birds Eye Inspirations 2 Pink Salmon Fillets with Lemon & Dill	280	154	3.9	0.1	4.00

Per 100g Rather Than Pack

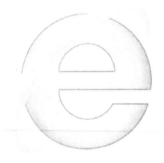

Find Us on the Web

WWW.WECANTSPELLSUCCESSWITHOUTYOU.COM

&

WWW.NADIET.INFO

Sardines

Suggested Brands	Size (g)	Kcal	S.fat (g)	Carbs (g)	£
Lusso Vita Sardine Fillets in Olive Oil & Lemon drained	80	165.6	0.2	0.3	1.79
Lusso Vita Sardine Fillets in Olive Oil & Chilli drained	80	165.6	0.2	0.3	1.79
Lusso Vita Skinless & Boneless Sardine Fillets in Olive Oil drained	84	173.9	0.3	0.3	1.79
ASDA Sardines in Tomato Sauce	106	127.2	0.7	1.3	1.00
Brunswick Sardines in Lousiana Hot Sauce	106	178.1	1.1	2.4	0.90
Tesco Skinless Boneless Sardines In Tomato Sauce	90	130.5	1.3	1.8	0.85
Morrisons Boneless Sardine Fillets with Lemon & Herb Dressing	100	109.0	1.4	1.5	0.82
Brunswick Sardines in Tabasco	106	133.6	1.4	0.0	0.90
Brunswick Sardines in Soya Oil	106	134.6	1.5	0.0	0.90
Tropical Sun Canadian Style Sardines in Spring Water	106	124.0	1.8	0.0	0.89
John West Boneless Sardines in Tomato Sauce	95	134.9	1.8	1.4	1.20
ASDA Sardines in Sunflower Oil	106	212.0	2.0	0.0	1.00

FISH   SARDINES

Suggested Brands	Size (g)	Kcal	S.fat (g)	Carbs (g)	£
Essential Waitrose sardines in sunflower oil drained	84	192.4	2.1	0.3	0.50
Waitrose sardine al limone drained	84	154.6	2.2	0.0	1.49
Morrisons Sardines In Tomato	120	174.0	2.3	1.6	0.40
Waitrose sardine fillets in olive oil drained	84	208.3	2.3	0.3	1.25
ASDA Sardines in Sunflower Oil	120	237.6	2.3	0.0	0.36
John West Sardines in Brine	120	207.6	2.8	0.0	1.00
Waitrose sardine piccanti drained	84	188.2	2.9	0.0	1.49
Hyacinthe Parmentier sardines in olive oil and chilli drained	95	217.6	2.9	0.0	1.99
Apollo Sardines In Vegetable Oil	125	288.8	2.9	0.0	0.80
John West Sardines in Tomato Sauce	120	196.8	3.0	1.8	1,00
M savers Sardines in Tomato Sauce	120	206.4	3.0	0.8	0.34
Riga Gold Brisling Sardines in Olive Oil with Chilli	120	242.4	3.0	1.4	1.50
Tesco Sardines In Brine	120	204.0	3.1	0.0	0.40
John West Sardines in Olive Oil	120	261.6	3.1	0.0	1.00
John West Boneless Sardines in Olive Oil	95	213.8	3.2	0.0	1.20

FISH SARDINES

Suggested Brands	Size (g)	Kcal	S.fat (g)	Carbs (g)	£
Hyacinthe Parmentier sardines in extra virgin olive oil drained	95	217.6	3.3	0.0	1.99
Hyacinthe Parmentier sardines in olive oil with herbs drained	95	217.6	3.3	0.0	1.99
Connétable MSC Sardines Extra Virgin Olive Oil drained	102	227.5	3.4	0.0	2.50
essential Waitrose Sardines in Olive Oil drained	84	252.0	3.4	0.4	0.52
John West Sardines in Sunflower Oil	120	261.6	3.4	0.0	1.00
Essential Waitrose sardines in water drained	84	165.5	3.5	0.5	0.50
Tesco Sardines In Tomato Sauce	120	210.0	3.5	1.1	0.40
Sainsbury's Sardines in Tomato Sauce	120	223.2	3.6	2.2	0.45
Sainsbury's Sardines in Brine	120	217.2	3.7	1.0	0.45
Morrisons Sardines In Brine	120	219.6	3.7	1.3	0.40
Sainsbury's Sardines in Chilli Oil	120	291.6	3.7	0.1	0.50
Tesco Sardines In Sunflower Oil	120	264.0	3.8	0.0	0.40
Lusso Vita Sardines Olive Oil with Slice of Lemon drained	95	287.9	3.8	0.0	1.49

FISH SARDINES

Suggested Brands	Size (g)	Kcal	S.fat (g)	Carbs (g)	£
Tropical Sun Sardines in Sunflower Oil with Chilli	125	286.3	3.9	0.5	0.74
Sainsbury's Sardines in Spring Water	120	234.0	4.1	1.4	0.50
ASDA Smart Price Sardines in Tomato Sauce	120	249.6	4.1	3.2	0.34
Morrisons The Best Sardines In Oil Infused Lemon Chilli & Garlic	105	278.3	4.1	1.4	0.70
Morrisons Sardines In Olive Oil	120	294.0	4.1	0.1	0.40
Hyacinthe Parmentier sardines in tomato sauce	135	199.8	4.2	4.2	1.99
Riga Gold Brisling Sardines in Olive Oil	120	255.6	4.2	0.0	1.50
Riga Gold Smoked Brisling Sardines in Olive Oil	120	255.6	4.2	0.0	1.50
Tesco Finest Sardines In Paprika And Tomato Sauce	105	293.0	4.3	1.2	0.90
Sainsbury's Sardines in Sunflower Oil	120	304.8	4.4	1.0	0.50
Morrisons The Best Sardines In Oil Infused With Sea Salt	105	282.5	4.5	0.1	0.87
Morrisons The Best Sardines In Oil Infused With Lemon	105	295.1	4.5	0.9	0.87
Tesco Finest Brisling Sardines In Water	105	239.4	4.6	0.2	0.90
Morrisons Sardines In Sunflower Oil	120	390.0	4.7	0.4	0.40

FISH   SARDINES

Suggested Brands	Size (g)	Kcal	S.fat (g)	Carbs (g)	£
Tesco Finest Sardines With Chilli, Lime And Coriander	105	302.4	4.8	0.6	0.90
Lusso Vita Sardines Olive Oil with Sundried Tomato	135	283.5	5.0	3.4	1.49
Parmentier Petites Sardines in Olive Oil drained	110	301.4	5.3	0.0	1.99
essential Waitrose sardines in tomato sauce	120	240.0	5.6	1.4	0.50
Parmentier Petites Sardines Olives in Olive Oil drained	110	299.2	5.6	1.5	1.99
Sainsbury's Sardines in Olive Oil	120	333.6	6.2	0.0	0.55

VALUES SHOWN PER TIN

Smoked Salmon

Suggested Brands	Size (g)	Kcal	S.fat (g)	Carbs (g)	£
Tesco Smoked Salmon Sushi	58	148	0.6	27.4	1.00
Waitrose wild Alaskan smoked salmon, 4 slices	100	126	0.7	1.2	6.99
Inverawe sliced Scottish smoked salmon	100	126	0.8	1.3	5.99
Formans Smoked Salmon Pellicle	100	168	0.8	0.05	3.75
H. Forman & Son Smoked Salmon	100	168	0.8	0.05	6.25
Sainsbury's Lemon & Pepper Smoked Salmon with Sicilian Lemon Oil	100	160	1.1	1.3	3.75
Tesco Finest Lemon And Pepper Smoked Salmon	120	164	1.1	3.4	4.80
Wild Smoked Sockeye Salmon	100	155	1.3	0.5	6.25
Leap Wild Alaskan Smoked Sockeye Salmon	100	155	1.3	0.5	6.39
ASDA Smoked Salmon	120	163	1.5	0.6	3.00
Sainsbury's Smoked Salmon Trimmings	100	176	1.5	1.4	2.50
Sainsbury's Scottish Smoked Salmon Sandwich Slices	100	196	1.5	1.1	3.75
Suempol Smoked Salmon	100	200	1.5	0.8	2.70
Waitrose Duchy Organic mild smoked salmon, 4 slices	120	156	1.6	0.05	6.99

FISH   SMOKED SALMON

Suggested Brands	Size (g)	Kcal	S.fat (g)	Carbs (g)	£
Connoisseur Norwegian Traditionally Smoked Salmon	100	166	1.6	0.0	3.00
Waitrose 1 Chestnut Smoked Scottish Salmon	100	176	1.6	0.6	5.99
Tesco 6 Smoked Salmon For Sandwiches	100	180	1.7	3.6	3.75
Tesco Finest Scottish Smoked Salmon	60	184	1.7	1.4	2.70
Tesco Finest Scottish Smoked Salmon	120	184	1.7	1.4	4.80
Tesco Smoked Salmon	120	185	1.7	1.5	3.00
Harbour Smokehouse Salmon	100	188	1.7	3.3	2.95
Sainsbury's Oak Smoked Scottish Salmon, Taste the Difference	100	196	1.8	0.9	4.35
Tesco Finest Gravadlax Smoked Salmon	160	213	1.8	7.8	4.80
Tesco Finest Counter Traditional Smoked Salmon Fillet	130	216	1.8	0.0	2.75
Waitrose Gin & Botanicals Smoked Salmon	100	185	1.9	2.5	4.49
ASDA Extra Special Rich & Intense Smoked Salmon	120	203	1.9	0.05	3.99
Waitrose 2 lightly smoked salmon fillets	240	179	2.0	0.0	5.24
Heston from Waitrose lapsang souchong tea smoked salmon, 4 slices	100	181	2.0	0.05	5.49

FISH   SMOKED SALMON

Suggested Brands	Size (g)	Kcal	S.fat (g)	Carbs (g)	£
ASDA Extra Special Mild & Delicate Smoked Salmon	120	200	2.0	0.05	3.99
Sainsbury's Mild Smoked Salmon	100	204	2.0	1.1	3.25
Bleiker's Traditional Oak Smoked Salmon	100	223	2.0	0.0	2.69
Grants Traditional Smoked Scottish Salmon	300	157	2.1	0.3	7.99
Tesco 2 Sweet Chill Hot Smoked Salmon Fillets	180	234	2.1	4.6	4.50
Morrisons 2 Lightly Smoked Salmon Fillets 2	240	238	2.1	0.5	5.00
Morrisons Hot Smoked Sweet Chili Salmon	180	241	2.1	2.8	4.00
Waitrose Hot Smoked Salmon with Sweet Chilli	160	247	2.1	4.5	5.00
Waitrose Scottish smoked salmon pieces	100	174	2.2	0.05	3.99
ASDA Smoked Salmon Trimmings	120	198	2.2	0.05	1.65
Morrisons The Best Scottish Smoked Salmon Slices	120	203	2.2	0.5	4.50
Sainsbury's Scottish Smoked Salmon with Dill & Mustard Dressing	130	211	2.2	3.9	4.25
2 Tandoori Spiced Hot Smoked Salmon Fillets	180	228	2.2	5.2	4.50
ASDA Kiln Roasted Salmon Flakes	120	235	2.2	0.8	3.50

Suggested Brands	Size (g)	Kcal	S.fat (g)	Carbs (g)	£
Scottish Monarch Smoked Scottish Salmon	90	157	2.3	0.3	2.09
Morrisons The Best Scottish Smoked Salmon With Treacle	120	226	2.3	6.8	5.00
Sainsbury's Salmon Fillet, Lightly Smoked, Taste the Difference x2	240	226	2.3	0.05	5.95
Sainsbury's Maple & Thyme Smoked Salmon Slices	150	234	2.3	2.7	4.50
Sainsbury's Hebridean Kiln Dried Smoked Salmon, Taste the Difference	100	229	2.4	0.05	3.85
Tesco Hot Smoked Salmon Fillets	180	234	2.4	1.1	4.50
ASDA Chipotle Chilli Roasted Salmon Fillets	180	258	2.4	1.9	3.99
Waitrose mild Scottish smoked salmon	100	184	2.7	0.05	4.99
ASDA Kiln Roasted Lemon & Parsley Salmon Fillets	180	251	2.7	2.9	3.99
Sainsbury's Gin & Juniper Smoked Salmon	100	243	2.9	1.0	3.95
Waitrose 1 Peat & Heather Scottish smoked salmon	100	173	3.0	0.05	5.99
Morrisons Hot Smoked Honey Roast Salmon Fillets 2 Pack	180	303	3.1	4.0	4.00

Suggested Brands	Size (g)	Kcal	S.fat (g)	Carbs (g)	£
John Ross Jr. Scottish smoked Scottish salmon	200	102	3.8	0.6	6.99
Morrisons Smoked Salmon	60	238	4.0	0.5	2.00
Ghillie & Glen Scottish smoked salmon minimum 6 slices	200	204	5.2	0.2	6.99
ASDA Extra Special 4 Smoked Salmon Stars	180	177	5.9	2.3	1.88
12 Smoked Salmon Canapes	100	241	6.1	4.1	3.00

Values Shown Per 100 Grams

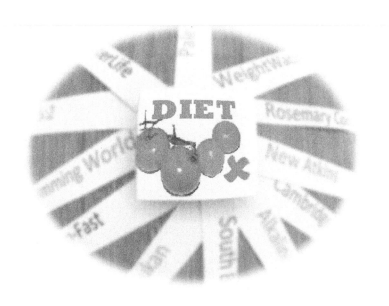

Tuna Steaks

Suggested Brands	Size (g)	Kcal	S.fat (g)	Carbs (g)	£
Ocean Ice Tuna Steaks	300	96.8	0.2	0.0	4.25
Iceland 4 Tuna Steaks	400	107.0	0.2	0.0	4.50
New England Seafood 2 Albacore Tuna Steaks	220	145.2	0.2	0.1	5.49
ASDA 2 Albacore Tuna Steaks	220	148.5	0.2	0.3	4.00
Morrisons Fishmongers Favourite Tuna Steaks X 4	360	90.0	0.3	0.0	3.30
Iceland The Fish Market 4 Tuna Steaks	400	100.0	0.3	0.0	4.00
Waitrose 1 fresh line-caught Tuna Steaks X 2	220	135.3	0.3	0.1	6.94
Tesco Tuna Steaks X 4	400	136.0	0.3	0.0	3.70
Wild Albacore Tuna Steaks X 2	220	162.8	0.3	0.1	5.50
ASDA 3 Yellowfin Tuna Steaks	270	112.5	0.4	0.0	3.15
Counter Tuna Steak X 4	420	123.9	0.4	0.5	10.50
Sainsbury's Tuna Steaks, Taste the Difference x2	240	148.8	0.4	0.1	6.50
Waitrose 1 yellowfin 2 tuna steaks X 2	240	166.8	0.4	0.1	7.99
ASDA Extra Special 2 Yellowfin Tuna Steaks	240	141.6	0.5	0.4	6.00
ASDA Extra Special 2 Yellowfin Tuna Loin Steaks	250	156.3	0.5	0.4	5.00

VALUES SHOWN PER STEAK

Notes

Meats

Always remember when choosing your meat:

You will find the most nutritious meat at the local butcher where it has escaped being processed. This meat will be more expensive than the supermarkets, but you will eat less in quantity as this type of meat is very filling when consumed. You will also benefit from being healthier due to eating a natural none processed product.

If you do not have a butcher's close to where you live or find them too expensive, you can purchase fresh meat for delivery using an online meat suppliers. These meats are a lot cheaper when purchased in bulk where only a small amount of the meat, if any, has been processed.

The cheapest meat is available at the local supermarket, this has generally been processed or ultra-processed, and is lower in nutritional value but higher in calories, fats and carbohydrates.

These types of meats are tasty when cooked and ate. The additional ingredients and additives, such as brine water, flour, sugar, sodium nitrite and potassium nitrate are added to the food that benefits the supermarkets profits rather than our health.

Bacon

Suggested Brands	Size (g)	Kcal	S.fat (g)	Carbs (g)	£
Sainsbury's Unsmoked Dry Cured British Bacon Medallions 160g, Taste the Difference x8	160	28.6	0.1	0.2	2.50
The Butcher's Market 10 Unsmoked Lean Bacon Medallions	250	27.8	0.2	0.1	2.00
The Butcher's Market 10 Smoked Lean Bacon Medallions	250	27.8	0.2	0.1	2.00
Quorn Meat Free Bacon Slices X 8	150	40.1	0.2	1.0	2.00
Morrisons Unsmoked Back Bacon Rashers 10 Pack	300	84.3	0.2	0.2	2.00
Morrisons Eat Smart Smoked Bacon x 8	248	49.0	0.3	1.1	2.00
Morrisons Eat Smart 8 Lean Unsmoked Bacon Medallions	248	48.7	0.4	0.3	2.00
Tesco Meat Free Bacon Style Rashers 8 Pack	150	63.9	0.4	1.0	1.75
Oakpark Unsmoked Bacon Medallions 6 Pack	170	38.3	0.6	0.3	2.00
Wall's Thick Cut Unsmoked Bacon 6 Rashers	146.8	37.0	0.7	0.2	2.00
Oakpark Smoked Bacon Medallions 6 Pack	170	40.8	0.7	0.3	2.00

MEATS   BACON

Suggested Brands	Size (g)	Kcal	S.fat (g)	Carbs (g)	£
Tesco Unsmoked 10 Medallions	300	46.8	0.7	0.0	2.85
ASDA Butcher's Selection 8 Reduced Fat Smoked Bacon Medallions	250	58.4	0.7	0.0	1.90
ASDA Butcher's Selection 8 Reduced Fat Unsmoked Bacon Medallions	250	66.6	0.9	0.0	1.90
Wall's Thick Cut Smoked Bacon 6 Rashers	146.8	41.6	1.0	0.2	2.00
ASDA Extra Special 16 Oak Smoked Dry Cured Streaky Bacon Rasher	240	46.5	1.1	0.1	2.20
Finnebrogue Smoked 12 Naked Streaky Bacon	200	44.0	1.2	0.1	3.00
Tesco Unsmoked Back Bacon Rasher x 10	300	54.0	1.2	0.1	1.50
Tesco Smoked Back Bacon Rashers x 10	300	54.0	1.2	0.1	1.50
J.James & Family Unsmoked Back Bacon Rashers x8	200	64.0	1.2	0.4	1.00
Tesco Finest Smoked Dry Cure Streaky Bacon x 16	240	48.5	1.3	0.2	2.50
J.James & Family Smoked Back Bacon Rashers x8	200	65.8	1.3	0.3	1.00
ASDA Extra Special 8 Dry Cured Unsmoked Back Bacon Rashers	240	70.8	1.3	0.0	2.20

MEATS BACON

Suggested Brands	Size (g)	Kcal	S.fat (g)	Carbs (g)	£
essential Waitrose smoked British thin cut back bacon, 10 rashers	200	43.6	1.4	0.0	2.00
Iceland 10 Rashers Average Smoked Back	300	57.0	1.4	0.2	2.00
Tesco Finest Unsmoked Wiltshire Cured Back Bacon 8 Pack	240	76.5	1.6	0.3	2.50
Sainsbury's Unsmoked Wiltshire Cured Back Bacon, Taste the Difference x8	240	78.0	1.6	0.0	2.00
Suffolk Crown Sweetcure Back Bacon x 8	200	69.3	1.7	0.3	2.00
Iceland 12 Smoked Streaky Bacon	270	57.8	1.8	0.1	2.00
Jolly Hog Oak & Beech Smoked Dry Cure Streaky Bacon x12	200	58.5	1.8	0.0	2.50
Waitrose smoked British streaky bacon, 12 rashers	250	59.6	1.8	0.0	3.49
Sizzlers Smoked Back Bacon Rasher x8	240	83.7	1.8	0.3	1.75
Sizzlers Unsmoked Back Bacon Rasher x8	240	83.7	1.8	0.3	1.75
Morrisons Smoked Back Bacon Rashers 10 Pack	300	84.3	1.8	0.2	2.00
Finnebrogue Unsmoked 6 Naked Back Bacon	200	85.7	1.8	0.3	3.00
Morrisons The Best Old Fashion Cure Bacon x 6	200	94.3	1.8	1.1	2.50

Suggested Brands	Size (g)	Kcal	S.fat (g)	Carbs (g)	£
Spoilt Pig Dry Cured Smoked Streaky Bacon x 10	184	66.8	1.9	0.0	3.14
Waitrose smoked British back bacon, 8 rashers	250	70.9	1.9	0.0	3.49
Waitrose unsmoked British back bacon, 8 rashers	250	70.9	1.9	0.0	3.49
Tesco Finest Smoked Wiltshire Cured Back Bacon 8 Pack	240	74.4	1.9	0.3	2.50
Iceland Luxury 6 Unsmoked Dry Cured Back Bacon	200	77.3	1.9	0.1	2.00
Finnebrogue Smoked 6 Naked Back Bacon	200	79.0	1.9	0.4	3.00
Tesco Smoked Streaky Bacon 14 Rashers	300	57.2	2.0	0.0	1.95
ASDA Butcher's Selection 10 Unsmoked Back Bacon Rashers	300	78.3	2.0	0.0	1.90
ASDA Butcher's Selection 10 Smoked Back Bacon Rashers	300	82.2	2.0	0.0	1.90
Sainsbury's Oak Smoked Wiltshire Cured Back Bacon, Taste the Difference x8	240	83.4	2.0	0.3	2.00
The Jolly Hog Unsmoked Back Bacon x 6	200	88.7	2.0	0.3	2.50

Suggested Brands	Size (g)	Kcal	S.fat (g)	Carbs (g)	£
The Jolly Hog Smoked Back Bacon x 6	200	88.7	2.0	0.3	2.50
The Jolly Hog Smoked Treacle Bacon x 6	200	89.0	2.0	0.8	2.50
Iceland 10 Rashers Average Unsmoked Back	300	66.3	2.1	0.2	2.00
Finnebrogue Unsmoked 12 Naked Streaky Bacon	200	67.2	2.1	0.3	3.00
Spoiltpig Smoked Dry Cured Back Bacon Rashers x 6	184	83.1	2.1	0.1	3.00
Sainsbury's Unsmoked Back Bacon Rashers x8	250	91.3	2.1	0.3	1.50
essential Waitrose smoked British streaky bacon, 12 rasher	250	56.0	2.2	0.0	2.00
essential Waitrose 10 British Outdoor Bred smoked back bacon rashers	300	65.4	2.2	0.0	2.39
Spoiltpig Unsmoked Dry Cured Back Bacon Rashers	184	73.3	2.2	0.2	3.00
Sainsbury's Reduced Salt Smoked Back Bacon x8	250	87.5	2.2	0.4	1.50
Morrisons The Best 6 Wiltshire Unsmoked Cured Back Bacon Rashers	200	93.7	2.2	0.2	2.50
Tesco Unsmoked Thick Cut Back Bacon x 6	300	85.0	2.4	0.0	1.95
Tesco Smoked Thick Cut Back Bacon x 6	300	85.0	2.4	0.0	1.95

MEATS   BACON

Suggested Brands	Size (g)	Kcal	S.fat (g)	Carbs (g)	£
Morrisons Extra Thick Unsmoked Back Bacon Rashers 6 Pack	300	115.5	2.4	0.3	2.00
Morrisons Smoked Extra Thick Rindless Back Bacon Rashers 6	300	115.5	2.4	0.3	2.00
Sainsbury's Oak Smoked Dry Cure Bacon, Taste the Difference x6	220	100.8	2.6	0.4	2.50
ASDA Farm Stores Unsmoked Back Bacon x 6	300	110.5	2.7	0.1	1.00
Sainsbury's Thick Unsmoked Back Bacon Rasher x4	200	116.5	2.7	0.5	1.80
Sainsbury's Thick Unsmoked Bacon Rasher x6	300	116.5	2.7	0.5	2.00
Sainsbury's Thick Smoked Bacon Rashers x6	300	116.5	2.7	0.5	2.00
Sainsbury's, Unsmoked Dry Cure Bacon, Taste the Difference x 6	220	104.5	2.8	0.4	2.50
Morrisons The Best Dry Cure Smoked Streaky Bacon x 8	240	115.8	3.1	0.4	2.50
essential Waitrose smoked British thick cut back bacon, 6 rashers	300	109.0	3.6	0.1	2.39
Sainsbury's Unsmoked Lean Bacon Loin Steaks x2	250	221.3	3.9	1.4	3.00

VALUES SHOWN PER SLICE

Beef Burger

Suggested Brands	Size (g)	Kcal	S.fat (g)	Carbs (g)	£
ASDA Meat Free 8 Beef Style Burgers	454	76.6	0.2	2.6	1.50
Tesco Meat Free Meat Style Burgers 8Pk	454	90.2	0.5	4.1	1.75
ASDA Butcher's Selection 4 Sea Salt & Pepper Turkey Burgers	454	166.8	1.6	3.6	2.70
Haloodies Beef Burgers 2oz X 6	340	151.3	1.9	4.9	2.75
Waitrose Reduced Fat British Beef Burger x 2	227	247.4	2.2	7.6	3.00
Morrisons Eat Smart 4 Beef Burgers	454	191.8	2.5	2.6	3.47
Slimming World Free Food 4 Syn-Free Beef Quarter Pounders	454	188.4	2.6	7.5	3.50
2 x Quorn Meat Free Classic Burger	180	163.8	2.9	8.8	2.50
Sainsbury's Chargrill Quarter Pounders, Be Good To Yourself x4	454	185.0	3.0	5.2	2.00
ASDA Smart Price 8 British Beef Burgers	397	120.6	3.1	6.5	1.30
Sainsbury's Beef Burgers, Basics x8	397	117.1	3.2	5.9	1.35
Sainsbury's Reduced Fat Burgers, Butcher's Choice x4	454	210.0	3.7	1.1	2.50

Suggested Brands	Size (g)	Kcal	S.fat (g)	Carbs (g)	£
Morrisons The Best 6Oz British Chuck Burgers x 4	340	169.2	4.0	2.0	3.00
ASDA 8 British Beef Burgers	454	147.0	4.1	4.2	2.00
ASDA 16 Beef Burgers	908	147.0	4.1	3.2	3.95
ASDA Butcher's Selection 4 Reduced Fat Beef Burgers	454	208.8	4.2	8.3	2.70
ASDA 4 Reduced Fat Quarter Pounder Beef Burgers	454	214.5	4.2	7.8	2.35
ASDA Extra Special 4 Seasoned Beef Burgers	454	204.3	4.4	6.1	3.00
Birds Eye 4 Original Beef Burgers With Onions	227	168.0	4.8	1.5	1.80
2 x The Beyond Burger	227	317.8	4.8	7.5	4.95
2 x Beyond Meat Free From Meat Burger	227	317.8	4.8	7.5	5.50
Tesco Beef Burgers 8 Pack	454	151.0	4.9	2.6	2.50
ASDA 4 Quarter Pounder Beef Burgers	264	174.2	4.9	5.0	2.00
Waitrose Duchy Organic 4 British beef burgers	340	198.9	4.9	2.5	4.25
ASDA Butcher's Selection 8 Beef Burgers	681	192.4	5.3	8.5	4.00
Tesco Finest 4 British Beef Steak Burgers	454	236.1	5.7	4.4	3.00
Sainsbury's Premium Beef Burger, SO Organic x2	228	249.7	5.8	5.5	2.50
Feasters 8 Flame Grilled Beef Burgers	440	155.1	5.9	1.4	3.00

MEATS BEEF BURGER

Suggested Brands	Size (g)	Kcal	S.fat (g)	Carbs (g)	£
DC Comics 4 Beef & Cheese Burgers	340	198.1	6.0	3.7	2.50
Tahira 12 Halal Chicken And Beef Burgers	780	171.6	6.1	6.5	3.50
Tesco Finest 4 Caramelised Onion Burger	454	253.1	6.1	8.4	3.00
Iceland 4 Beef Smokehouse Quarter Pounders	454	242.9	6.5	8.3	2.00
essential Waitrose 4 quarter pounders 100% British beef	454	255.4	6.5	0.1	2.79
Waitrose Frozen 4 Aberdeen Angus beef quarter pounders	454	255.4	6.5	0.1	3.59
DC Comics 4 Beef, Cheese & Bacon Burgers	340	212.5	6.7	3.2	2.50
ASDA Butcher's Selection 4 Quarter Pounder Beef Burgers	454	256.5	7.0	11.4	2.49
Feasters Microwave Cheese Burger	147	379.3	7.5	33.8	1.00
ASDA Extra Special 4 Caramelised Pink Onion Beef Burgers	454	274.7	7.6	7.6	3.00
Iceland 4 Quarter Pounders X 4	454	266.7	7.7	6.1	1.85
Morrisons The Best Steak Hache Burgers x 2	340	382.5	7.7	2.4	3.00
DC Comics 4 Beef Burgers	340	231.2	7.8	4.8	2.50

MEATS   BEEF BURGER

Suggested Brands	Size (g)	Kcal	S.fat (g)	Carbs (g)	£
Waitrose 4 Aberdeen Angus beef quarter pounders	454	297.4	7.8	4.0	4.30
ASDA Extra Special 2 Aberdeen Angus Beef Steak Burgers	340	362.1	8.0	5.4	3.00
ASDA Butcher's Selection 4 Red Onion & Cheese Beef Burgers	454	274.7	8.1	7.2	2.70
Waitrose 4 Applewood Beef Burgers	454	305.3	8.2	4.5	4.00
Sainsbury's Beef Burgers With Caramelised Onion, Taste the Difference x2	340	367.2	8.3	13.3	2.50
Sainsbury's Beef Burgers, Butcher's Choice x4	454	281.5	8.4	4.2	2.50
Iceland Luxury 4 Aberdeen Angus Quarter Pounders	454	280.3	8.5	0.6	2,25
Morrisons 4 Beef Quarter Pounders with Onions	454	284.9	8.5	4.3	2.35
Morrisons The Best Scotch Beef Quarter Pounders	454	286.0	8.5	2.8	3.00
ASDA 4 Bacon & Cheese British Beef Quarter Pounders	454	287.2	8.5	7.2	2.00
Tesco Finest 2 Gluten Free Beef Burgers	340	353.6	8.5	6.6	2.50
ASDA Extra Special 2 Wagyu Beef Burgers	340	377.4	8.5	4.3	4.00
Tesco 4 1/4Lb Beef Burgers	454	279.2	8.7	7.0	2.00

Suggested Brands	Size (g)	Kcal	S.fat (g)	Carbs (g)	£
Morrisons 4 Beef Quarter Pounders with Cheese	454	283.8	8.7	4.5	2.35
ASDA Extra Special 4 Aberdeen Angus Beef Quarter Pounders x 4	454	301.9	8.9	4.4	2.50
Rustlers Flame Grilled Beef Burger	156	405.6	8.9	42.4	2.00
Tariq Halal Beef Burger x 4	450	266.6	9.0	2.3	3.50
Iceland 4 Double Cheeseburgers	454	263.3	9.1	5.2	2.25
Iceland Luxury 2 Aberdeen Angus Beef Burgers	284	313.8	9.5	4.8	2.00
J.James & Family Beef & Pork Hamburgers x4	454	334.8	9.5	4.0	1.90
Birds Eye 4 Original Beef Quarter Pounders	454	336.0	9.5	3.1	3.00
Sainsbury's Beef Quarter Pounders x4	454	305.3	9.6	2.7	2.30
Gourmet Burger Kitchen 2 British beef burgers	342	384.8	9.7	0.2	3.00
Haloodies Quarter Pounder Beef Burgers X 2	227	303.0	9.8	3.9	1.75
ASDA 4 Indian Spiced Beef Quarter Pounders	454	303.0	10.1	4.3	2.00
Morrisons The Best 4 Vintage Cheddar Beef Burgers	454	325.7	10.1	3.4	3.00
2 x Tesco Cheese Burgers In Buns	505	595.9	10.1	63.6	3.15
ASDA 4 Quarter Pounder Beef Burgers	454	323.5	10.2	1.5	2.35

Suggested Brands	Size (g)	Kcal	S.fat (g)	Carbs (g)	£
Iceland 4 100% British Beef Quarter Pounders	454	339.4	10.8	0.0	2.00
Birds Eye 4 Inspirations Mozzarella, Sundried Tomato & Basil Beef Quarter Pounders	454	362.1	10.9	3.0	3.29
Tesco Finest Beef Burger 6Oz	170	374.0	11.6	3.2	1.30
Iceland Luxury 2 Ultimate 5oz Steak Burgers	284	380.6	11.6	1.6	2.25
Sainsbury's Beef Burgers With West Country Cheddar, Taste the Difference x2	340	402.9	11.7	4.4	2.50
Tesco Finest 4 British Beef Burgers	454	342.8	12.0	0.6	3.00
Sainsbury's British Beef Burgers, Taste the Difference x2	340	425.0	13.4	3.1	2.50
Birds Eye Inspirations 2 5oz Beef Steak Burgers	284	475.7	13.9	2.1	2.50
Shazan Select HMC Beef Burgers x 4	454	398.4	14.2	5.9	3.50
Waitrose 2 Highland beef burgers	340	470.9	15.8	3.6	4.99

VALUES SHOWN PER BURGER

Boiled Ham

Suggested Brands	Size (g)	Kcal	S.fat (g)	Carbs (g)	£
Iceland 7(Average) Breaded Ham Slices	120	106	0.4	2.0	1.39
Iceland 7 Slices (Average) Cooked Ham	120	104	0.5	1.3	1.39
Henry Denny & Sons 8 Slices Crumbed Ham	90	97	0.6	1.0	1.00
Sainsbury's Ham Finely Sliced, Be Good To Yourself	100	98	0.6	0.2	1.75
Quorn Vegan Smoky Ham Free Slices	100	101	0.6	1.7	2.00
ASDA Thin Bavarian Smoked Ham Slices	140	102	0.6	0.2	1.65
Morrisons Carvery Smoked Ham	170	107	0.6	1.5	2.00
Morrisons Carvery Thinly Sliced Honey Roast Ham	155	110	0.6	1.9	2.00
ASDA Thick Dry Cured Honey Roast Ham Slices x 4	150	117	0.6	2.3	1.65
ASDA Finely Sliced Honey Roast Dry Cured Ham	150	117	0.6	2.3	1.65
Sainsbury's Finely Sliced Honey Roast Yorkshire Ham, Taste the Difference	120	118	0.6	1.8	2.70
ASDA Cooked Ham Slices	300	99	0.7	2.8	1.50
Iceland 7(Average) Peppered Ham Slices	120	113	0.7	1.3	1.39

MEATS   BOILED HAM

Suggested Brands	Size (g)	Kcal	S.fat (g)	Carbs (g)	£
ASDA Finely Sliced Oak Smoked Dry Cured Ham	150	113	0.7	1.9	1.65
Iceland 7(Average) Honey Roast Ham Slices	120	117	0.7	2.0	1.39
Morrisons The Best Finely Sliced Applewood Smoked Ham	100	123	0.7	1.2	2.35
Morrisons The Best Thick Cut Honey Roast Ham	120	133	0.7	2.7	2.35
Tesco The Deli Family Pack Crumbed Ham Slices	425	102	0.8	1.3	4.00
Finnebrogue Naked Deli Ham Slices	500	105	0.8	1.3	2.00
ASDA Finely Sliced Oven Baked Dry Cured Ham	150	114	0.8	1.8	1.79
ASDA Thick Dry Cured Ham Slices	150	114	0.8	1.8	1.79
ASDA Thick Sliced Oven Baked Dry Cured Ham	500	115	0.8	1.8	4.50
Sainsbury's British Cooked Ham Wafer Thin Sliced	400	101	0.9	1.2	2.00
Sainsbury's Wafer Thin Cooked Ham	70	102	0.9	1.0	0.55
Sainsbury's British Honey Cured Ham Wafer Thin Sliced	400	114	0.9	3.6	2.00
Houghton Cooked Sliced Northampton Ham	130	116	0.9	0.7	2.79
Tesco Finest Wiltshire Finely Sliced Ham	125	119	0.9	0.2	3.00

Suggested Brands	Size (g)	Kcal	S.fat (g)	Carbs (g)	£
Iceland 30 Cooked Ham Slices	350	102	1.0	0.0	1.89
Morrisons Wafer Thin Smoked Ham Slices	400	102	1.0	1.8	2.00
Morrisons Wafer Thin Honey Roast Ham Slices	400	105	1.0	2.9	2.00
Deli Co Crumbed Lean Ham 14 Slices	300	107	1.0	2.5	1.59
Waitrose British ham, 6 slices	120	111	1.00	0.0	2.99
Waitrose British honey roast ham, 6 slices	120	117	1.0	0.0	2.99
Fire & Smoke Louisiana Style Fire Grilled Ham Slices	100	137	1.0	1.0	2.00
Fire & Smoke Slow Cooked Fire Grilled Ham	100	137	1.0	1.0	2.22
ASDA Thick Breaded Dry Cured Ham Slices	150	123	1.1	1.8	1.65
Iceland Luxury 100% British Pork Finely Sliced Dry Cured Cooked Ham	100	131	1.1	3.3	1.79
Quorn Vegetarian Ham Slices	100	123	1.2	5.2	1.60
Bernard Matthews Turkey Ham Wafer Thin	380	110	1.3	3.7	2.50
ASDA Finely Sliced BBQ Dry Cured Ham	150	135	1.3	2.4	1.75
Iceland Luxury Finely Sliced Applewood Smoked Ham	100	141	1.3	3.2	1.79

MEATS   BOILED HAM

Suggested Brands	Size (g)	Kcal	S.fat (g)	Carbs (g)	£
essential Waitrose British Ham 8 Slices	100	116	1.4	0.2	1.65
ASDA Extra Special Hand Breaded Wiltshire Ham Slices	130	131	1.4	0.2	2.50
Sainsbury's British Thick Cut Wiltshire Cured Ham, Taste the Difference	120	133	1.4	0.2	2.70
Fire & Smoke Bourbon Smoked Fire Grilled Ham	100	141	1.4	1.5	2.22
Waitrose British oak smoked ham, 6 slices	120	130	1.5	0.0	2.99
Morrisons Deli Breaded Ham Slices	160	133	1.5	2.9	2.00
Waitrose British Wiltshire Cured Breaded Ham 4 Slices	130	135	1.5	0.9	3.49
Morrisons The Best Finely Sliced Honey Roast Dry Cured Ham	100	147	1.5	2.7	2.35
ASDA Cooked Ham Slices	200	107	1.6	0.2	1.20
Waitrose German smoked Brunswick ham, 6 slices	120	130	1.6	0.5	2.69
Waitrose British Wiltshire Cured Ham 4 Slices	130	134	1.6	0.1	3.49
Iceland Luxury 4 Slices Breaded Wiltshire Ham	100	144	1.8	0.8	1.79
ASDA Wafer Thin Cooked Ham	400	126	2.1	1.0	1.85
ASDA Smart Price Cooked Ham Slices	400	112	2.2	0.2	1.29

Suggested Brands	Size (g)	Kcal	S.fat (g)	Carbs (g)	£
ASDA Smart Price Wafer Thin Cooked Ham Slices	400	112	2.2	0.2	1.49
Waitrose British Wiltshire Thick Cut Cured Ham 3 Slices	130	152	2.2	0.1	3.49
ASDA Wafer Thin Smoked Ham Slices	200	117	2.3	0.2	1.00
ASDA Wafer Thin Honey Roast Ham Slices	200	128	2.4	3.1	1.00
ASDA Wafer Thin Honey Roast Ham	400	129	2.4	3.1	1.85
Iceland Luxury Finely Sliced Honey Roast Ham	100	166	2.5	3.2	1.79
VBites Cheatin Ham Style Slices	100	234	4.8	4.3	1.70

VALUES SHOWN PER 100 GRAMS

Chicken Burger

Suggested Brands	Size (g)	Kcal	S.fat (g)	Carbs (g)	£
Quorn chicken style x4	252	129.2	0.6	10.4	2.00
Birds Eye 4 Chicken	200	121.5	0.7	10.0	1.00
Morrisons 2 Southern Fried Fillet	250	261.3	0.9	18.0	2.50
Iceland 10 Breaded Chicken	550	138.1	1.1	10.2	2.00
ASDA 10 Breaded Golden Chicken	570	164.7	1.1	10.3	2.08
Fry's Meat Free 4 Chicken Style	320	157.6	1.2	9.7	2.95
ASDA 4 Buttermilk Chicken Breast Fillet	400	195.0	1.3	11.0	2.50
ASDA Smart Price 8 Breaded	456	159.0	1.4	11.4	0.97
Heck Simply Chicken x2	228	124.3	1.5	3.8	2.50
Hearty Food Co 8 Breaded	456	155.0	1.5	11.0	0.97
Tesco 4 Southern Fried Chicken	380	204.3	1.7	11.5	1.50
Feasters Microwave Southern Fried Chicken	130	322.4	2.1	39.5	1.00
Birds Eye 2 Chicken Quarter Pounders	227	303.1	2.2	20.5	1.00
Speedy Snacks Chicken Burger	142	353.6	2.3	43.2	1.00
Rustlers Southern Fried Chicken Burger with Our Lightly Peppered Mayo	145	410.4	2.3	39.7	1.00
Morrisons 8 Chicken Burgers	456	200.1	2.7	11.2	1.70

MEATS CHICKEN BURGER

Suggested Brands	Size (g)	Kcal	S.fat (g)	Carbs (g)	£
Sainsbury's Breaded British Chicken x2	460	503.7	2.8	33.4	2.00
Sainsbury's Chicken Quarter x4	454	181.6	2.9	6.5	2.50
Sainsbury's Chicken Burgers x2	456	335.2	3.2	12.6	2.00

VALUES SHOWN PER BURGER

Your Favourite Food Not Included?
Let Us Know

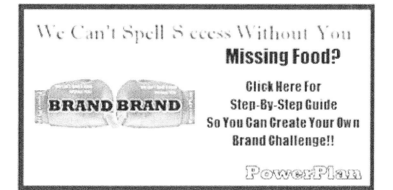

WWW.WECANTSPELLSUCCESSWITHOUTYOU.COM

Chicken Fillet

Suggested Brands	Size (g)	Kcal	S.fat (g)	Carbs (g)	£
Tesco Finest 2 Cornfed Free Range Chicken Fillets	320	105	0.2	1.0	4.39
M Organic Free Range Chicken Breast Fillets	275	131	0.2	0.0	4.68
Tesco Organic 2 Chicken Fillets	320	104	0.3	0.0	6.92
The Butcher's Market Class 'A' Chicken Breast Fillets	500	106	0.3	0.0	2.00
Tesco 2 British Chicken Breast Fillets	300	106	0.3	0.0	2.50
Valley Foods Skinless Chicken Fillets	500	115	0.4	0.1	2.50
Waitrose 1 Free Range 2 chicken breast fillets	300	130	0.4	0.1	5.40
Morrisons Chicken Fillets	700	133	0.4	0.5	3.25
ASDA Butcher's Selection Chicken Breast Fillets	1000	138	0.4	0.0	5.79
Waitrose Duchy Organic 2 Free Range British chicken breast	300	144	0.4	0.1	6.82
Butchers Choice Chicken Breast Fillets	1000	92	0.5	0.2	3.50
Azeem Halal Chicken Breast Fillets	1000	94	0.5	0.3	4.00
Iceland Ready Cooked Sliced Chicken Breast	500	120	0.5	0.8	3.00

Suggested Brands	Size (g)	Kcal	S.fat (g)	Carbs (g)	£
Sainsbury's Free Range Chicken Breast Fillets, SO Organic	1000	131	0.5	0.1	20.95
ASDA Butcher's Selection Chicken Breast Fillet	300	132	0.5	0.1	1.80
ASDA Butcher's Selection Chicken Breast	650	132	0.5	0.1	3.80
ASDA Butcher's Selection Chicken Breast Fillet Portions	525	132	0.5	0.1	4.00
Sainsbury's Free Range Chicken Breast Fillets, Taste the Difference x2	1000	136	0.5	0.1	18.00
Sainsbury's Chicken Breast Fillets	320	137	0.5	0.1	2.40
Sainsbury's British Skinless Chicken Fillets	1000	137	0.5	0.2	5.25
ASDA Cook from Frozen Chicken Breast Fillets	1000	124	0.6	0.2	4.99
Tesco Chicken Breast Fillet	1000	128	0.6	0.4	5.50
Morrisons Chicken Breast Fillet	630	131	0.6	0.0	4.00
essential Waitrose 3-5 British chicken breast fillets	500	140	0.6	0.1	3.95
essential Waitrose British chicken breast fillets	1000	140	0.6	0.1	9.80
Waitrose Omega 3 chicken breast fillets	490	141	0.6	0.0	7.84

MEATS   CHICKEN FILLET

Suggested Brands	Size (g)	Kcal	S.fat (g)	Carbs (g)	£
Morrisons The Best Corn Fed Free Range Chicken Breast Fillets	340	138	0.7	0.0	4.92
The Butcher's Market Chicken Breast Fillets	1150	128	0.8	0.8	5.00
Morrisons Savers Chicken Fillets	1000	126	0.9	0.5	3.65
Hank & Joes Chicken Fillets	1500	134	0.9	0.1	6.00
Shazans Halal Chicken Breast Fillets	450	116	1.1	0.1	4.00
Shazan Select HMC Small Chicken Breast Fillet	450	116	1.1	0.2	4.00
ASDA Smart Price Chicken Breast Fillets	1000	152	1.1	0.2	3.50
ASDA Farm Stores Chicken Breast Fillet Portions	620	159	1.2	0.1	3.09
Tesco Finest British Cornfed Free Range Skin On Chicken Fillets	340	136	1.6	0.0	4.66

VALUES SHOWN PER 100 GRAMS

Chicken Nugget

Suggested Brands	Size (g)	Kcal	S.fat (g)	Carbs (g)	£
Quorn Crispy Nuggets x 15	300	32.2	0.1	3.2	2.00
Iceland 32 Breaded Chicken Nuggets	448	35.8	0.2	25.6	1.50
ASDA 34 Battered Chicken Nuggets	600	39.5	0.2	3.7	2.00
Ella's Kitchen Big Kids Starry Chicken Nuggets X 8	200	48.0	0.2	6.0	3.50
ASDA Smart Price 20 Breaded Chicken Nugget	320	42.2	0.3	3.2	0.89
Birds Eye 24 Chicken Nuggets	379	42.5	0.3	3.3	3.00
Birds Eye 50 Chicken Nuggets with Golden Wholegrain	790	42.5	0.3	3.3	3.75
ASDA 34 Breaded Chicken Nuggets	600	43.1	0.3	2.6	1.89
Tesco Meat Free Chicken Style Nuggets 16 Pack	320	46.6	0.3	3.9	1.75
Birds Eye Gluten Free Chicken Nuggets x 22	455	52.5	0.3	4.3	3.75
Tesco 30 Breaded Chicken Nuggets	450	38.7	0.4	2.6	1.50
Morrisons 62 Breaded Chicken Nuggets	1000	43.2	0.4	3.1	3.15
Morrisons 62 Breaded Chicken Nuggets	1000	43.2	0.4	3.1	3.15
Hearty Food Co 20 Breaded Chicken Nuggets	320	44.5	0.4	3.9	0.89

MEATS   CHICKEN NUGGET

Suggested Brands	Size (g)	Kcal	S.fat (g)	Carbs (g)	£
Tesco Free From 20 Chicken Nuggets	400	50.8	0.5	3.1	3.50
Tesco 20 Battered Chicken Dippers	450	64.1	0.7	3.9	1.50
Aishas Value Chicken Nuggets X 20	500	69.3	0.7	4.7	2.00

VALUES SHOWN PER SLICE

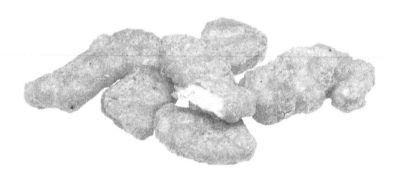

Gammon Joint

Suggested Brands	Size (g)	Kcal	S.fat (g)	Carbs (g)	£
Sainsbury's Honey Glazed Gammon Joint	800	238.0	1.0	7.0	5.50
Morrisons Eat Smart Unsmoked Gammon	700	211.8	1.1	0.4	4.00
Morrisons Smoked Gammon Joint	750	189.4	1.7	0.6	3.20
Morrisons Smoked Gammon Joint	750	189.4	1.7	0.6	3.20
ASDA Butcher's Selection Smoked Gammon Joint	750	196.9	1.7	0.4	2.65
Tesco Roast In Bag Unsmoked Gammon Joint	840	237.3	1.7	1.1	5.00
Dalehead Roast in the Bag Unsmoked Gammon (Serves 3)	500	273.3	1.7	0.0	4.99
Waitrose Unsmoked Gammon Joint	570	195.2	1.9	0.0	5.70
ASDA Butcher's Selection Unsmoked Gammon Joint	750	198.8	1.9	0.4	2.65
Morrisons Gammon With Honey Glaze	600	219.0	2.1	1.5	3.00
ASDA Simple to Cook Honey and Maple Gammon Joint	700	248.5	2.3	1.6	4.25
Morrisons Unsmoked Gammon Joint	750	208.1	2.4	0.2	3.20
Iceland Smoked Gammon Joint serves 5	1000	210.0	2.4	0.0	4.00

MEATS GAMMON JOINT

Suggested Brands	Size (g)	Kcal	S.fat (g)	Carbs (g)	£
Iceland Unsmoked Gammon Joint serves 5	1000	210.0	2.4	0.0	4.00
Tesco Gammon Joint With Honey (Serves 3)	550	331.8	2.9	13.4	3.50
Morrisons Plain Cook In The Bag Gammon Joint	700	206.5	3.2	0.4	4.00
British Outdoor Bred Unsmoked Gammon Joint, Taste the Difference	750	309.4	3.6	3.2	7.50
Morrisons Maple Glaze Cook In The Bag Gammon Joint	700	241.5	4.4	0.5	4.00
Sainsbury's Unsmoked Gammon Joint	750	320.6	4.7	1.9	3.60
Sainsbury's Smoked Gammon Joint	750	320.6	4.7	1.9	3.60
Iceland Roast From Frozen Easy Carve Boneless Basted Gammon Joint with a Honey Glaze	700	337.8	5.4	3.5	3.00
Sainsbury's Just Cook Honey Gammon Joint 470g (Serves 3)	470	308.6	6.3	3.3	4.00
Sainsbury's Just Cook British Gammon Joint With Apple & Blackberry Glaze (Serves 3)	470	319.6	6.9	6.4	3.75
Waitrose Easy To Cook Gammon joint with a sweet maple syrup glaze (Serves 3)	456	381.5	8.8	7.8	5.99

VALUES SHOWN PER SERVING

Liver

Suggested Brands	Size (g)	Kcal	S.fat (g)	Carbs (g)	£
Waitrose Duchy Organic chicken livers	400	82	0.3	0.4	2.69
Counter Pork Liver	380	106	1.0	0.3	1.20
Counter Chicken Liver	380	106	1.0	0.3	1.20
Counter Lamb Liver	500	159	1.1	4	1.20
Counter Ox Liver	380	165	1.4	3.8	1.20
Banham Poultry Chicken Livers	225	233	2.0	0.1	0.50
essential Waitrose British Chicken Livers	400	146	2.1	0.9	1.15
ASDA Chicken Livers	227	186	2.9	0.1	0.90
Waitrose Omega 3 chicken livers	400	166	3.4	1.3	1.28

VALUES SHOWN PER 100 GRAMS

Mince

Suggested Brands	Size (g)	Kcal	S.fat (g)	Carbs (g)	£
Meat the alternative beef style mince made with soya	500	133.5	0.2	10.4	2.99
ASDA Butcher's Selection Extra Lean Turkey Mince (Typically Less Than 3% Fat)	500	211.5	0.5	0.1	3.49
Sainsbury's Turkey Breast Mince 2% Fat	500	204.0	0.6	0.0	4.35
Quorn Meat Free Mince	500	156.0	0.8	6.8	3.00

Meats Mince

Suggested Brands	Size (g)	Kcal	S.fat (g)	Carbs (g)	£
Morrisons Market St Turkey Breast Mince	500	168.0	0.8	0.2	4.00
essential Waitrose British Turkey Breast Mince	300	214.5	0.8	0.2	4.00
Morrisons Meat Free Mince	400	187.5	1.2	5.7	1.50
Sainsbury's British Pork Mince 5% Fat	500	199.5	1.4	0.0	2.20
Sainsbury's Vegetarian Mince	500	211.5	1.5	10.1	1.75
ASDA Meat Free Mince	454	268.5	1.7	12.2	1.50
Sainsbury's British Turkey Thigh Mince 7% Fat	500	219.0	1.8	3.3	2.00
The Butcher's Market Scottish Lean Beef Steak Mince Typically 5% Fat	400	163.5	2.3	0.0	3.00
The Butcher's Market British Lean Beef Steak Mince Typically 5% Fat	400	163.5	2.3	0.0	3.00
Waitrose Venison Mince	300	178.5	2.4	0.1	4.50
ASDA Extra Special Aberdeen Angus Beef Mince (Typically Less Than 5% Fat)	500	196.5	2.4	0.1	3.75
Waitrose Pork Lean Mince Typically 5% Fat	500	192.0	2.6	0.0	3.00
ASDA Butcher's Selection Lean Pork Mince (Typically Less Than 5% Fat)	500	246.0	2.6	1.2	3.00
The Butcher's Market Pork Mince 20% Fat	500	249.0	2.6	0.0	2.00

MEATS MINCE

Suggested Brands	Size (g)	Kcal	S.fat (g)	Carbs (g)	£
Tesco Pork Lean Mince 5% Fat	500	189.0	2.7	0.0	3.00
ASDA Butcher's Selection Lean Beef Mince (Typically Less Than 5% Fat)	500	225.0	2.7	0.1	2.97
ASDA Butcher's Selection Lean Turkey Mince (Typically Less Than 7% Fat)	500	210.0	2.9	0.1	2.25
Morrisons British Minced Pork 5% Fat	500	268.5	2.9	0.0	3.00
Tesco Beef Lean Steak Mince	500	186.0	3.0	13.5	3.30
Sainsbury's Beef Mince 5% Fat, SO Organic	400	249.0	3.2	0.1	3.80
Sainsbury's 5% Fat Beef Mince	500	250.5	3.2	0.1	3.75
Sainsbury's Beef Mince 5% Fat	500	252.0	3.2	0.1	3.10
Iceland Lean Steak Mince	475	177.0	3.3	0.0	3.00
Waitrose Aberdeen Angus lean mince beef, 5% fat	400	187.5	3.3	0.0	5.00
essential Waitrose British Turkey Thigh Mince	500	283.5	3.5	0.2	3.65
Tesco Lean Beef Steak Mince 5 % Fat	500	196.5	3.6	0.5	3.75
ASDA Lean Turkey Mince	500	289.5	3.9	0.1	2.50
essential Waitrose British Beef Lean Mince	500	214.5	4.7	0.0	3.65
essential Waitrose British pork mince	500	226.5	5.0	0.1	2.30

MEATS   MINCE

Suggested Brands	Size (g)	Kcal	S.fat (g)	Carbs (g)	£
Waitrose Duchy free range British pork mince	500	226.5	5.0	0.1	4.19
Woodside Farms 12% Fat Pork Mince	500	268.5	6.2	0.0	2.20
Tesco Healthy Living 10% Fat Minced Beef Steak	500	262.5	6.5	0.0	3.50
Naked Glory Mince	260	270.0	6.6	13.5	2.00
essential Waitrose British mince beef, 10% fat	500	255.0	6.8	0.0	3.20
Waitrose Frozen Hereford beef mince	500	255.0	6.8	0.0	3.99
Waitrose Duchy Organic British lean beef mince, 10% fat	400	255.0	6.8	0.0	4.30
Waitrose Aberdeen Angus mince beef, 10% fat	400	255.0	6.8	0.0	4.30
Waitrose Hereford lean beef mince, 10% fat	400	255.0	6.8	0.0	4.30
ASDA Reduced Fat Beef Mince	800	289.5	6.8	0.1	3.50
Sainsbury's Lamb Mince 10% Fat	500	288.0	6.9	0.1	5.50
ASDA Butcher's Selection Reduced Fat Beef Mince (Typically Less Than 12% Fat)	500	301.5	7.1	3.6	2.09
Sainsbury's British Pork Mince 10% Fat	500	363.0	7.7	0.9	2.10
Iceland Beef Steak Mince	550	255.0	8.1	0.0	3.00
The Butcher's Market Beef Steak Mince	1100	255.0	8.1	0.0	5.00

Suggested Brands	Size (g)	Kcal	S.fat (g)	Carbs (g)	£
Sainsbury's Beef Mince 12% Fat	500	309.0	8.1	0.1	2.60
Sainsbury's Beef Mince 12% Fat, SO Organic	400	309.0	8.1	0.1	3.00
Sainsbury's Beef Mince 12% Fat, Taste the Difference	500	312.0	8.3	0.1	3.50
Morrisons Market St British Minced Beef 12 % Fat	500	285.0	8.4	0.0	2.35
Morrisons The Best Matured Scotch Beef Mince 12% Fat	500	285.0	8.4	0.0	3.50
ASDA Butcher's Selection Lamb Mince (Typically Less Than 20% Fat)	500	318.0	8.6	2.0	3.20
ASDA Butcher's Selection Pork Mince (Typically Less Than 20% Fat)	500	387.0	9.6	4.2	1.99
Tesco Beef Steak Mince 15% Fat	500	313.5	9.8	0.0	2.50
Tesco Finest Aberdeen Angus Steak Mince	500	313.5	9.8	0.0	4.00
Tesco Organic Beef Steak Mince 15% Fat	500	313.5	9.8	0.0	4.65
Sainsbury's British Pork Mince 20% Fat	500	397.5	9.8	1.5	1.75
essential Waitrose British beef mince, 15% fat	500	328.5	10.1	0.0	2.75
Waitrose Aberdeen Angus Beef Mince 15% Fat	400	328.5	10.1	0.0	4.00

MEATS   MINCE

Suggested Brands	Size (g)	Kcal	S.fat (g)	Carbs (g)	£
Waitrose British Veal Mince	400	328.5	10.1	0.0	4.29
ASDA Butcher's Selection Beef Mince (Typically Less Than 20% Fat)	500	361.5	10.4	0.1	1.59
The Butcher's Market Beef Mince	1300	322.5	11.0	0.0	5.00
Morrisons British Minced Pork 20% Fat	500	385.5	11.0	0.0	2.10
Morrisons British Minced Beef 20% Fat	500	379.5	11.3	0.0	1.60
Iceland Lamb Mince	450	312.0	11.9	0.0	3.00
The Butcher's Market Lamb Mince	900	312.0	11.9	0.0	5.00
Naturli Pea Based Minced	400	315.0	11.9	14.4	3.00
Morrisons British Minced Lamb	500	352.5	12.8	0.0	4.00
Sainsbury's Beef Mince 20% Fat	500	409.5	12.8	1.2	1.65
Iceland Beef Pork & Mince	375	409.5	13.1	0.8	1.59
Boswell Farms Beef Mince 20% Fat	500	378.0	14.7	0.0	1.49
essential Waitrose British lamb mince 20% fat	500	370.5	15.3	0.2	4.49
Sainsbury's Lamb Mince 20% Fat	500	403.5	15.3	0.1	4.50
Sainsbury's Lamb Mince, SO Organic	400	403.5	15.3	0.1	4.80
The Butcher's Market British Beef Mince Typically 23% Fat	500	418.5	15.6	0.0	2.00

MEATS MINCE

Suggested Brands	Size (g)	Kcal	S.fat (g)	Carbs (g)	£
J.James & Family 25% Fat Beef & Pork Mince	750	475.5	15.8	0.1	2.75
Morrisons Minced Lamb	500	406.5	16.1	0.6	2.75
Sainsbury's New Zealand Lamb Mince	500	462.0	16.2	0.0	3.75
ASDA Beef Mince	800	388.5	16.5	5.7	3.20
ASDA Prime Cuts Lamb Mince	500	424.5	16.5	1.1	3.30
M savers Beef & Pork Mince	1000	448.5	17.0	0.2	3.20
The Butcher's Market British Beef Steak Mince Typically 12% Fat	500	928.5	28.5	0.1	2.89
The Butcher's Market Scottish Beef Steak Mince Typically 12% Fat	500	928.5	28.5	0.1	2.89

VALUES SHOWN PER 150 GRAMS

Pork Loin Steak

Suggested Brands	Size (g)	Kcal	S.fat (g)	Carbs (g)	£
Morrisons The Best Hampshire Pork Loin Medallions x 6	300	52.5	0.3	0.3	3.00
ASDA Butchers Selection British Pork Lean Loin Medallions x 6	450	114.8	0.8	0.8	3.09
ASDA Butcher's Selection Unsmoked Bacon Loin Steaks	400	178.0	2.0	1.0	2.50
ASDA Butcher's Selection Smoked Bacon Loin Steaks x 4	400	176.0	2.1	1.0	2.50
Morrisons Market Street British Pork Loin Medallions x 4	380	139.7	2.2	0.0	3.25
Morrisons British Pork Loin Steaks With Arrabiata Marinade x 4	400	213.0	3.3	1.4	4.00
Iceland 6 Salt & Chilli Pork Loin Steaks	440	189.2	4.1	2.3	2.50
Waitrose Easy To Cook 2 Pork loin medallions with cauliflower cheese melt & onion crumb	300	289.5	4.2	16.5	4.19
Sainsbury's Chinese Style British Pork Loin Steaks, Summer Edition x4	500	267.5	4.3	4.0	4.50
ASDA Butcher's Selection 4 Chinese Pork Loin Steaks	440	268.4	5.0	3.7	3.00

MEATS PORK LOIN STEAK

Suggested Brands	Size (g)	Kcal	S.fat (g)	Carbs (g)	£
Sainsbury's British Pork Loin Steaks x4	480	262.8	5.2	1.3	2.80
The Butcher's Market 8 Pork Loin Steaks	1000	261.3	5.4	0.0	5.00
Tesco Thin Cut Pork Loin Steaks 6 Pack	600	225.0	5.9	0.0	3.50
essential Waitrose British thin cut pork loin steaks x 6	450	202.5	6.0	0.0	4.00
Waitrose Duchy Organic British free range pork loin steaks x 5	400	216.0	6.4	0.0	4.80
Sainsbury's Just Cook British Pork Loin Steaks With Sage & Onion Rub x2	250	293.8	6.4	3.0	2.75
Morrisons British Pork Loin Steaks x 4	500	281.3	7.4	0.0	3.00
Tesco Bbq Maple Pork Loin Steaks x 6	600	284.0	7.4	8.6	4.00
ASDA Prime Cuts 4 Pork Loin Steaks	600	373.5	7.7	4.1	3.30
Tesco Pork Loin Steaks 2 Pack	270	303.8	8.0	0.0	2.00
ASDA Butcher's Selection 6 Caribbean Pork Loin Steaks	660	298.1	8.1	4.1	4.00
ASDA Butcher's Selection Pork Loin Steaks x 4	480	362.4	8.9	0.2	2.10
Tesco Finest Pork Loin Steaks x 2	400	450.0	11.8	0.0	3.50

MEATS   PORK LOIN STEAK

Suggested Brands	Size (g)	Kcal	S.fat (g)	Carbs (g)	£
essential Waitrose British pork loin steaks x 2	300	405.0	12.0	0.0	1.85

VALUES SHOWN PER STEAK

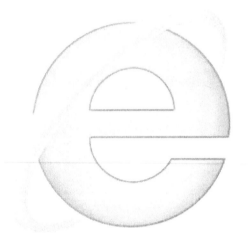

Find Us on The Web

WWW.WECANTSPELLSUCCESSWITHOUTYOU.COM

&

WWW.NADIET.INFO

Pork Spare Ribs

Suggested Brands	Size (g)	Kcal	S.fat (g)	Carbs (g)	£
Appleby's Smoky BBQ Ribs	600	1122	14.4	102	2.99
BBQ Pork Ribs Home Cooked From Raw	600	864	19.2	14.4	2.50
ASDA Ultimate Bourbon Boneless Beef Ribs	300	825	20.1	30	2.00
Waitrose slow cooked pork rack	535	1262.6	25.1	32.1	5.00
ASDA Hot & Spicy Pork Rack of Ribs	600	1422	28.8	52.2	3.75
Tesco BBQ Bourbon Glazed	460	1285.3	31.3	31.1	3.50
Morrisons Market St Hoi Sin Rack	550	1391.5	31.4	43.5	4.00
Morrisons Market St Smoky BBQ Rack	550	1545.5	31.4	41.8	4.00
ASDA Smoky BBQ Rack of Pork Ribs	600	1584	35.4	60	3.75
Sainsbury's Slow Cook Smokey BBQ	676	1865.8	37.9	58.8	5.00
Tesco Slow Cooked BBQ Maple Pork Ribs	460	1407.6	38.7	27.1	3.50
Sainsbury's Kansas Style BBQ	600	1668	42.6	37.8	5.00

Roast Duck

Suggested Brands	Size (g)	Kcal	S.fat (g)	Carbs (g)	£
ASDA Extra Special	2100	199	2.4	0.2	7.00
Gressingham British Whole Duck	2000	238	4.2	2.9	10.00

VALUES SHOWN PER 100 GRAMS UNCOOKED

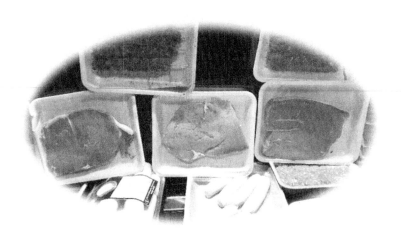

Sausages

Suggested Brands	Size (g)	Kcal	S.fat (g)	Carbs (g)	£
Linda McCartney's Meat Free 6 Red Onion & Rosemary Sausages	300	71.5	0.2	3.5	2.00
Linda Mccartney 6 Vegetarian Red Onion And Rosemary Sausages	300	71.5	0.2	3.5	2.00
HECK 10 Spring Chicken Sausages	340	49.6	0.3	0.4	2.50
Quorn Meat Free 6 Low Fat Sausages	300	63.0	0.3	4.4	1.70
HECK 10 Chicken Italia Sausages	340	49.3	0.4	0.8	2.98
Quorn Meat Free 8 Sausages	336	83.2	0.6	4.5	1.70
Slimming World Free Food 6 Pork, Squash & Sage Sausages	360	73.8	0.7	2.8	3.00
ASDA 8 Reduced Fat Pork Sausages	400	75.5	0.7	5.5	2.40
ASDA Extra Special 6 Light & Lean Pork Sausages	400	81.3	0.7	2.9	2.50
Powters 6 low fat sausages	400	96.7	0.9	6.9	3.09
Linda McCartney's Meat Free 6 Vegetarian Sausage	300	80.0	1.0	3.8	2.00
ASDA Butcher's Selection 8 Reduced Fat Pork Sausages	400	82.5	1.2	4.4	1.45

MEATS SAUSAGES

Suggested Brands	Size (g)	Kcal	S.fat (g)	Carbs (g)	£
Slimming World 6 pork sausages	360	92.4	1.3	0.5	3.00
Linda Mccartney 6 Vegetarian Sausages	300	120.0	1.4	5.6	2.00
ASDA Smart Price 20 Sausages	907	92.5	1.5	7.3	0.91
Tesco British Chicken Sausages 6 Pack	400	116.7	1.5	5.6	2.20
Butcher's Choice 20 Pork Sausages	907	98.0	1.6	6.7	0.91
Richmond 8 Chicken Sausages	400	103.0	1.7	7.0	2.50
Richmond 12 Thin Pork Sausages	340	76.2	1.9	4.5	1.60
Tesco 8 Reduced Fat Pork Sausages	454	109.5	1.9	4.3	1.70
Richmond 16 Skinless Frozen Pork Sausages	426	73.5	2.0	3.7	2.00
Morrisons Butchers Style Reduced Fat Pork Sausage	454	114.6	2.0	6.4	1.65
Morrisons Butchers Style Reduced Fat Cumberland Pork Sausage	454	115.8	2.0	6.1	1.65
Tesco Thick Pork And Beef Sausages 20 Pack	900	102.2	2.3	6.1	2.75
Tesco Reduced Fat Cumberland Sausage	454	118.6	2.3	8.2	1.70
Waitrose 8 Cumberland Sausages	454	130.0	2.3	3.6	2.79

MEATS SAUSAGES

Suggested Brands	Size (g)	Kcal	S.fat (g)	Carbs (g)	£
Ballineen Chip Shop Style 6 Cooked Irish Sausages in a Crispy Batter	240	146.4	2.3	12.4	1.50
ASDA Butcher's Selection 8 Pork Sausages	454	115.2	2.4	3.9	1.45
ASDA Butcher's Selection 12 Pork Sausages	681	115.2	2.4	3.9	2.09
Debbie And Andrews Pork Sausages x 10	600	92.4	2.6	1.9	3.00
Tesco 20 Cumberland Sausages	900	108.0	2.6	5.6	2.75
Tesco Thick Pork Sausages 20 Pack	900	112.1	2.7	5.2	2.75
ASDA Farm Stores 8 Pork Sausages	454	124.9	2.7	3.4	1.00
ASDA Butcher's Selection 8 Cumberland Sausages	454	116.9	2.8	3.4	1.45
ASDA 20 Thick Pork Sausages	1000	125.0	2.8	5.5	2.00
Mr Brain's 4 Pork Sausages in Our Classic West Country Sauce	409	506.2	2.8	9.2	1.25
ASDA Butcher's Selection 8 Pork & Apple	454	127.1	3.0	5.6	1.45
Waitrose 8 Lincolnshire Sausages	454	133.9	3.0	3.4	2.79
Sainsbury's Butcher's Choice Pork Sausages x8	454	135.6	3.0	6.8	1.50
Richmond 24 Thick Frozen Pork Sausages	1080	121.1	3.1	7.2	3.50

MEATS   SAUSAGES

Suggested Brands	Size (g)	Kcal	S.fat (g)	Carbs (g)	£
Richmond 14 Thick Frozen Pork Sausages	634	121.8	3.1	7.2	2.00
ASDA 20 Irish Recipe Pork Sausages	1000	132.0	3.2	6.0	2.00
Sainsbury's Butcher's Choice Cumberland Pork Sausages x8	454	142.4	3.2	5.3	1.50
Tesco British Lincolnshire Sausages 8 Pack	454	144.7	3.2	5.2	1.70
Wall's Ready Baked Pork Sausages x 6	275	127.9	3.3	6.9	2.00
Iceland 16 Thick Irish Recipe Pork Sausages	800	132.5	3.3	4.7	1.75
Herta Frankfurter Hot Dogs x10	350	99.8	3.4	0.7	1.75
ASDA Extra Special 6 Pork Welsh Cheddar & Smoked Bacon	400	111.5	3.4	1.3	2.15
Iceland 16 Pork & Beef Sausages	800	130.5	3.4	3.6	1.75
Sainsbury's Butcher's Choice Lincolnshire Pork Sausages x8	454	139.6	3.4	4.8	1.50
ASDA Butcher's Selection 8 Lincolnshire Sausages	454	132.2	3.5	1.1	1.45
Musk's 6 Gluten Free pork sausages	384	134.4	3.5	2.2	3.00
Powters 6 gluten-free sausages	400	141.3	3.5	0.0	3.09

Suggested Brands	Size (g)	Kcal	S.fat (g)	Carbs (g)	£
Waitrose Duchy Organic 6 British free range pork sausages with mixed herbs	400	147.3	3.5	1.3	2.84
Musk's 6 Newmarket pork sausages	384	148.5	3.5	4.9	3.05
ASDA 12 Cumberland Sausages	600	133.0	3.6	3.9	2.40
Walls Classic 8 Pork Sausages	454	137.9	3.6	3.9	2.10
Morrisons Butcher's Style Pork Sausages X 8	454	150.4	3.7	5.9	1.65
Morrisons Butcher's Style Thick Cumberland Sausages X 8	454	157.2	3.8	6.0	1.65
Plumtree Farms 40 Value Sausages	1800	135.9	3.9	2.7	2.00
Richmond 12 Thick Pork Sausages	681	152.7	3.9	9.1	3.20
Morrisons Butcher's Style Thick Lincolnshire Sausages X 8	454	160.0	3.9	5.7	1.65
Waitrose 6 British gourmet pork sausages with black pepper & nutmeg	400	168.7	3.9	3.9	3.29
Waitrose 6 British pork sausages with fresh leeks & chives	400	160.0	4.0	3.6	3.29
Iceland 8 British Thick Pork Sausages	454	162.3	4.0	4.9	1.69

MEATS SAUSAGES

Suggested Brands	Size (g)	Kcal	S.fat (g)	Carbs (g)	£
Tesco British Pork Sausages 8 Pack	454	170.8	4.1	5.1	1.70
Tesco Finest 6 British Pork And Caramelised Onion Sausages	400	166.0	4.2	6.2	2.50
Waitrose 6 British pork sausages with bramley apple	400	170.7	4.3	5.8	3.29
Powters 6 cider & sage sausages	400	171.3	4.3	8.4	3.09
Iceland Luxury 6 Cumberland Sausages	400	150.5	4.5	1.6	2.00
Henry Denny & Sons Gold Medal 8 Thick Pork Sausages	454	168.0	4.7	6.4	2.00
essential Waitrose British Pork 8 Sausages	454	168.0	4.8	4.9	1.98
Tesco British Cumberland Sausages 8 Pack	454	185.0	4.8	5.1	1.70
ASDA Extra Special 6 Lincolnshire Pork Sausages	400	170.0	4.9	1.7	2.15
ASDA Extra Special 6 Pork & Three Chilli Sausages	400	170.7	5.0	1.7	2.15
ASDA Extra Special 6 Pork Sausages	400	172.7	5.1	1.5	2.15
Waitrose 6 British pork sausages with caramelised red onion	400	201.3	5.1	4.2	3.29
Powters celebrated Newmarket sausages X 6	400	188.7	5.2	11.0	3.09

MEATS SAUSAGES

Suggested Brands	Size (g)	Kcal	S.fat (g)	Carbs (g)	£
Morrisons 8 Free From Sausages	454	181.0	5.4	2.9	2.00
ASDA Extra Special 6 Bacon & Maple Syrup	400	192.0	5.5	3.7	2.15
Tesco Finest 6 British Pork Bramley Apple Sausages	400	195.3	5.5	3.6	2.50
Iceland Luxury 6 Thick Pork Sausages	400	195.3	5.7	1.6	2.00
Tesco Finest 10 Traditional Pork Sausages	667	202.1	5.7	0.4	4.00
Waitrose 1 British free range Cumberland pork sausages 6s	400	212.0	5.7	0.9	3.29
Waitrose 1 free range 6 pork sausages	400	215.3	6.0	0.7	3.29
Tesco Finest British 6 Lincolnshire Sausages	400	196.0	6.1	0.4	2.50
Waitrose 1 British free range Lincolnshire pork sausages 6s	400	222.7	6.3	1.1	3.29
Tesco Finest 6 British Pork Cumberland Sausages	400	225.3	6.7	1.1	2.50
HECK 6 97% Pork Sausages	400	157.3	8.8	0.5	2.98

Values Shown Per Sausage Serving

Sauces (Cooking)

We all love a good curry, pasta bake or a spaghetti bolognese where we add a jar of sauce to the cooked onion, vegetables, meat or fish. We feel that we are cooking a good, nutritious healthy meal without realising the sauce can be calorific, high in fat and sugar. It is so easy to purchase the wrong sauce when trying to improve our health when cooking food at home. This results in undesirable weight and fitness results that are disappointing over time.

When using the following section, and switching to the correct sauce for your health needs, you will see a BIG difference in your life as your weight, health issues and fitness improves.

Consider looking at simple recipes so you can make your own sauces. Simply using canned tomatoes, water, garlic granules and BBQ spice with salt and pepper. This makes a wonderful alternative sauce for pasta or spaghetti bolognese dish. If you prefer a curry, use canned tomatoes, water, mild curry and turmeric spices with salt and pepper. This makes a wonderful alternative sauce for a curry dish.

Bolognese

Suggested Brands	Size (g)	Kcal	S.fat (g)	Carbs (g)	£
Homepride Bolognese Cooking Sauce	485	229.5	0.2	39.2	1.50
ASDA Calorie Counted Bolognese	500	165	0.3	31.5	0.75
Tesco No Added Sugar Bolognese	500	171.5	0.3	27	0.65
Tesco Bolognese Pasta Sauce	500	204.5	0.3	33	0.65
Ragu Original Smooth Bolognese	650	312	0.3	65.7	2.69
Mr Organic Bolognese	350	126	0.4	17.9	2.49
Morrisons Savers Pasta Sauce	440	154	0.4	20.7	0.42
ASDA Smart Price Bolognese	440	176	0.4	33.4	0.39
Morrison's Bolognese Sauce	500	180	0.5	28	0.83
Dolmio Bolognese Pasta Sauce	500	225	0.5	39.5	1.75
ASDA Extra Special Bolognese	340	173.4	1.0	18.4	1.09
Seeds Of Change Bolognese Organic	500	230	1.0	36.5	2.40
Loyd Grossman Bolognese Pasta Sauce	425	233.8	1.3	25.9	1.98
Waitrose suggo alla Bolognese	555	455.1	5.0	27.2	2.80

Butter Chicken

Suggested Brands	Size (g)	Kcal	S.fat (g)	Carbs (g)	£
Kohinoor Delhi Butter Chicken	375	490.1	4.9	46.5	1.89
Sharwood's Butter Chicken Mild Curry	420	424.2	11.3	31.5	1.84
Spice Tailor Classic Butter Chicken	300	363.0	12.3	26.7	2.90
Patak's Butter Chicken Curry	450	580.5	16.7	36.9	1.00
Sainsbury's Butter Chicken	500	505.0	19.5	36.5	0.65
Tesco Butter Chicken Sauce	500	535.0	20.0	34.5	0.75
ASDA Butter Chicken Curry	495	589.1	23.3	39.1	0.79

VALUES SHOWN PER FULL JAR

Chinese Curry

Suggested Brands	Size (g)	Kcal	S.fat (g)	Carbs (g)	£
Sharwood's Chinese Medium Curry Cooking Sauce	425	216.8	0.9	33.2	2.00
ASDA Curry Cooking Sauce	500	455.0	5.5	55.0	0.75
Sainsbury's Chinese Chip Shop Curry Sauce	500	350.0	7.5	38.0	0.65
ASDA Chinese Curry Cooking Sauce	500	380.0	8.5	42.5	0.79
Waitrose Katsu Curry Cooking	350	336.0	14.0	24.5	1.60

VALUES SHOWN PER FULL JAR

Your Favourite Food Not Included?
Let Us Know

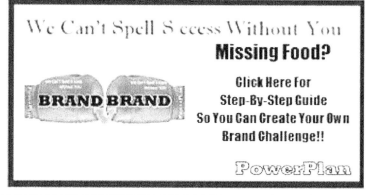

We Can't Spell S ccess Without You

Missing Food?

**Click Here For
Step-By-Step Guide
So You Can Create Your Own
Brand Challenge!!**

BRAND BRAND

PowerPlan

WWW.WECANTSPELLSUCCESSWITHOUTYOU.COM

Hunters Chicken

Suggested Brands	Size (g)	Kcal	S.fat (g)	Carbs (g)	£
ASDA Calorie Counted Hunter's Chicken Cooking Sauce	500	215.0	0.1	38.5	0.75
Homepride Hunter's Chicken Cooking Sauce	485	519.0	0.2	118.8	1.50
ASDA Hunters Chicken Cooking Sauce	515	360.5	0.3	82.4	0.84
Sainsbury's Hunters Chicken	530	487.6	0.3	109.7	0.65
Morrisons Hunters' Chicken Sauce	535	417.3	0.5	92.6	0.85
Tesco Hunters Chicken Cooking Sauce	515	458.4	1.0	100.4	0.75

VALUES SHOWN PER FULL JAR

Jalfrezi Curry

Suggested Brands	Size (g)	Kcal	S.fat (g)	Carbs (g)	£
Slimming World Free Food Jalfrezi	350	119.0	0.4	15.8	1.50
Sainsbury's Jalfrezi Sauce	500	270.0	1.0	29.5	0.65
Morrisons Jalfrezi Sauce	450	283.5	1.4	31.1	0.85
Tesco Jalfrezi Sauce	500	285.0	1.5	35.5	0.75
Sharwood's Jalfrezi Hot Curry Cooking Sauce	420	336.0	1.7	26.0	1.84
Bay's Kitchen Jalfrezi Curry	260	202.8	1.8	19.2	4.15
Tesco Finest Jalfrezi Cooking Sauce	350	252.0	3.9	24.9	1.59
Patak's Jalfrezi Curry Sauce	450	436.5	4.1	38.3	1.00
ASDA Jalfrezi Curry Sauce	500	395.0	4.5	49.0	0.79
East End Jalfrezi Curry Cooking	375	405.0	4.5	36.0	1.25
Kohinoor Delhi Butter Chicken Cooking Sauce	375	490.1	4.9	46.5	1.89
Patak's The Original Sizzle & Spice Jalfrezi Sauce	360	388.8	5.4	41.8	2.19
Geeta's Jalfrezi Spice & Stir	250	237.5	6.0	19.0	2.09
Loyd Grossman Jalfrezi Curry Sauce	350	318.5	6.0	25.6	1.00

VALUES SHOWN PER FULL JAR

Korma Curry

Suggested Brands	Size (g)	Kcal	S.fat (g)	Carbs (g)	£
Meridian Free From Korma Curry	350	283.5	14.7	27.7	1.85
Waitrose half fat korma	350	385.0	15.4	31.2	1.69
Sainsbury's Korma Light	500	440.0	17.5	47.0	0.65
ASDA Korma Spice & Simmer	360	439.2	18.4	26.3	0.99
Patak's The Original Sizzle & Spice Korma	360	460.8	18.7	40.7	2.19
Uncle Ben's Korma	450	513.0	18.9	46.8	1.88
Tesco Korma Sauce	500	440.0	19.0	48.5	0.75
Sharwood's Korma Reduced Fat	420	403.2	19.7	38.6	1.84
Loyd Grossman Korma	350	448.0	20.3	39.6	1.00
Seeds of Change organic Indian korma	350	483.0	21.7	34.3	2.40
Sharwood's Korma Mild Curry	420	525.0	24.4	45.4	1.84
Waitrose korma	350	696.5	26.6	42.7	1.69
Patak's Korma Curry	450	652.5	27.5	42.3	1.00
Tesco Finest Royal Korma	350	532.0	28.4	35.4	1.59
Morrisons Korma Sauce	450	688.5	32.0	37.8	0.85
Sainsbury's Korma Sauce	500	705.0	39.0	46.5	0.65
ASDA Korma Curry	500	955.0	49.5	47.5	0.79

VALUES SHOWN PER FULL JAR

Pasta Bake

Suggested Brands	Size (g)	Kcal	S.fat (g)	Carbs (g)	£
ASDA Tomato & Garlic Pasta Sauce	500	210.0	0.1	39.0	0.64
Dolmio Lasagne Sauce Red Tomato	500	230.0	0.1	45.0	1.75
ASDA Bolognese Pasta Sauce	500	175.0	1.0	29.5	0.64
ASDA Spicy Tomato Pasta Sauce	500	215.0	1.0	33.5	0.64
ASDA Red Lasagne Sauce	500	215.0	1.0	35.0	0.64
ASDA Tomato & Chunky Vegetable Pasta Sauce	500	230.0	1.0	37.0	0.64
Dolmio Mediterranean Vegetable Pasta Bake Sauce	500	260.0	1.0	40.5	1.75
Homepride Pasta Bake Tomato, Garlic & Chilli	485	514.1	2.4	46.1	1.50
Homepride Pasta Bake Creamy Tuna	485	417.1	2.9	34.9	1.50
Homepride Pasta Bake Tomato & Herb	485	504.4	3.4	34.9	1.50
Homepride Pasta Bake Spicy Tomato & Pepperoni	485	388.0	3.9	43.2	1.50
ASDA Tomato and Bacon Pasta Bake	480	408.0	4.3	37.0	0.75
Dolmio Tomato & Cheese Pasta Bake	500	290.0	4.5	42.5	1.75
ASDA Chilli Cheese Pasta Bake	495	485.1	4.5	49.5	0.79

SAUCES (COOKING) PASTA BAKE

Suggested Brands	Size (g)	Kcal	S.fat (g)	Carbs (g)	£
Sainsbury's Pasta Bake Sauce Spicy Pepperoni	510	515.1	4.6	40.8	0.65
Homepride Pasta Bake Cheese & Bacon	485	378.3	5.3	20.9	1.50
ASDA Tuna Pasta Bake Cooking Sauce	480	585.6	5.3	38.4	0.79
ASDA Spicy Tomato & Pepperoni Pasta Bake	500	555.0	5.5	47.5	0.79
ASDA Cheese & Bacon Pasta Bake	480	441.6	5.8	34.6	0.75
Tesco Pasta Bake Creamy Tomato And Herb	500	405.0	6.0	27.0	0.75
Homepride Pasta Bake Tomato & Bacon	485	509.3	6.3	34.9	1.50
Tesco Free From Tom And Basil Bake	500	420.0	7.5	38.5	1.30
Dolmio Creamy Tomato Pasta Bake	500	450.0	8.5	44.0	1.75
Homepride Pasta Bake Cheesy	485	465.6	9.2	27.6	1.50
Sainsbury's Creamy Tomato Pasta Bake	480	633.6	11.0	35.5	0.65
ASDA Creamy Tomato Pasta Bake	500	650.0	12.5	29.0	0.75
essential Waitrose creamy tomato pasta bake	555	333.0	13.3	26.6	1.55
ASDA Macaroni Cheese Pasta Bake	485	674.2	13.6	39.8	0.79
Sainsbury's Pasta Bake Sauce Macaroni Cheese	485	722.7	14.1	33.5	0.65

Suggested Brands	Size (g)	Kcal	S.fat (g)	Carbs (g)	£
Tesco Mac & Cheese Pasta Bake Sauce	460	611.8	15.2	29.4	0.85
Dolmio Carbonara Pasta Bake Sauce	480	595.2	15.8	25.4	1.75

VALUES SHOWN PER FULL JAR

Saag Curry

Suggested Brands	Size (g)	Kcal	S.fat (g)	Carbs (g)	£
Indi Grand Saag Curry	375	371.3	1.1	48.8	0.60
Patak's Saag Masala	450	315.0	3.2	24.8	1.89
Sharwood's Tika Malasa with Saag Curry	420	411.6	13.9	37.4	1.84

VALUES SHOWN PER FULL JAR

Sausage Casserole

Suggested Brands	Size (g)	Kcal	S.fat (g)	Carbs (g)	£
Morrisons Sausage Casserole	500	205.0	0.0	45.0	0.85
Homepride Sausage Casserole	485	194.0	0.2	41.2	1.50
ASDA Sausage Casserole Cooking Sauce	500	340.0	0.3	60.0	0.75

VALUES SHOWN PER FULL JAR

Stir Fry

Suggested Brands	Size (g)	Kcal	S.fat (g)	Carbs (g)	£
Celebrate Health Recipe Base Chinese Beef	175	99.8	0.0	4.9	1.59
Celebrate Health Recipe Base Teriyaki	175	222.3	0.0	11.6	1.59
Blue Dragon Oyster & Spring Onion	120	124.8	0.1	29.2	0.60
Blue Dragon Teriyaki	120	138.0	0.1	32.3	0.60
ASDA Sweet & Sour	170	151.3	0.1	34.0	0.80
ASDA Sweet & Sour	120	156.0	0.1	37.2	0.35
Blue Dragon Sweet & Sour	120	158.4	0.1	39.2	0.60
Blue Dragon Chinese BBQ	120	184.8	0.1	43.6	0.60
Blue Dragon Sweet Chilli & Garlic	120	190.8	0.1	39.4	0.60
Blue Dragon Chow Mein	150	241.5	0.1	57.0	1.30
Tesco Hoi Sin	120	110.4	0.2	22.7	0.50
Blue Dragon Chow Mein	120	127.2	0.2	27.6	0.60
ASDA Sweet Chilli	170	136.0	0.2	30.6	0.80
ASDA Sweet Chilli & Garlic	120	145.2	0.2	32.4	0.39
Tesco Plum And Hoisin	180	174.6	0.2	39.6	1.00
ASDA Hoi Sin	170	178.5	0.2	34.0	0.80
Amoy Sweet Thai Chilli	120	187.2	0.2	45.5	0.99
Tesco Teriyaki	180	201.6	0.2	43.6	1.00
Tesco Chinese	180	111.6	0.3	16.6	1.00
Tesco Sweet Chilli	180	199.8	0.3	42.8	1.00
ASDA Chow Mein	120	91.2	0.4	16.8	0.35
ASDA Hoisin	120	103.2	0.4	21.6	0.35
ASDA Black Bean	120	124.8	0.4	22.8	0.39
ASDA Szechuan	120	134.4	0.4	25.2	0.39
Blue Dragon Black Bean	120	148.8	0.4	28.3	0.60

Suggested Brands	Size (g)	Kcal	S.fat (g)	Carbs (g)	£
Blue Dragon Hoisin & Garlic	120	176.4	0.4	37.8	0.60
Tesco Sweet And Sour	180	230.4	0.4	44.3	1.00
ASDA Blackbean	170	159.8	0.5	20.4	0.80
Amoy Black Bean	120	115.2	0.6	16.9	0.99
Amoy Chow Mein	120	164.4	0.8	25.3	0.99
ASDA Soy & Garlic	170	178.5	0.9	28.9	0.80
ASDA Chow Mein	170	202.3	1.5	20.4	0.80
Blue Dragon Satay	150	346.5	3.2	55.5	1.30
ASDA Satay	120	202.8	4.0	16.8	0.39
Amoy Peanut Satay	120	217.2	5.4	20.3	0.99
Tesco Coconut And Lemon Grass	180	147.1	8.5	9.7	1.00

Sweet And Sour

Suggested Brands	Size (g)	Kcal	S.fat (g)	Carbs (g)	£
Uncle Ben's Sweet & Sour No Added Sugar	440	136.4	0.0	24.2	1.88
ASDA Smart Price Sweet & Sour	440	228.8	0.0	53.2	0.34
Sainsbury's Lighter Sweet & Sour	500	265.0	0.0	57.0	0.65
Sainsbury's Sweet & Sour	500	285.0	0.0	64.5	0.65
ASDA Sweet & Sour Cooking Sauce	500	350.0	0.0	85.0	0.69
Uncle Ben's Sweet and Sour	450	360.0	0.0	73.8	1.88

SAUCES (COOKING)   SWEET AND SOUR

Suggested Brands	Size (g)	Kcal	S.fat (g)	Carbs (g)	£
Uncle Ben's Sweet and Sour Extra Pineapple	450	369.0	0.0	76.1	1.88
ASDA Free From Sweet & Sour	500	380.0	0.0	85.0	1.50
Tesco Sweet And Sour Sauce	500	385.0	0.0	92.0	0.80
Sainsbury's Extra Pineapple Sweet & Sour	500	390.0	0.0	88.0	0.65
Sainsbury's Sweet & Sour Sauce, Basics	500	280.0	0.1	65.5	0.55
Seeds of Change Organic Sweet & Sour Sauce	350	343.0	0.2	80.5	1.50
Sharwood's 30% Less Sugar Sweet & Sour	425	284.8	0.4	60.8	1.74
essential Waitrose sweet & sour	500	445.0	0.5	103.0	0.95

VALUES SHOWN PER FULL JAR

Tikka Masala

Suggested Brands	Size (g)	Kcal	S.fat (g)	Carbs (g)	£
Iceland Luxury Tikka Masala Spice, Sizzle & Stir	360	356.4	2.9	22.7	1.25
Tesco Tikka Masala Cooking Sauce	500	370.0	3.5	44.5	0.75
Patak's Tikka Masala Indian Curry Sauce	450	364.5	3.6	32.9	1.00
Morrisons Tikka Masala Sauce	450	346.5	4.1	37.4	0.85
Uncle Ben's Tikka Masala Sauce	450	391.5	4.5	41.4	1.78
Tesco Hot Tikka Masala Cooking Sauce	500	450.0	4.5	54.5	0.75
ASDA Tikka Masala Spice & Simmer Curry Sauce	360	252.0	6.1	26.3	0.99
ASDA Tikka Masala Curry Sauce	500	400.0	6.5	55.0	0.69
Meridian Free From Tikka Masala Cooking Sauce	350	343.0	6.7	37.5	1.87
Sainsbury's Tikka Masala Light Sauce, Be Good To Yourself	500	380.0	8.5	46.5	0.65
Patak's The Original Sizzle & Spice Tikka Masala Sauce	360	439.2	8.6	39.6	2.19
ASDA Free From Tikka Masala Sauce	500	415.0	9.0	60.0	1.50
Seeds Of Change Tikka Masala Organic	350	413.0	9.8	29.4	2.40

Suggested Brands	Size (g)	Kcal	S.fat (g)	Carbs (g)	£
Sharwoods Tikka Masala 30% Less Fat Cooking Sauce	420	352.8	10.5	39.1	1.75
Sharwood's Tikka Masala Reduced Fat Curry Sauce	420	352.8	10.5	39.1	1.84
Sainsbury's Tikka Masala Sauce	500	525.0	11.0	50.5	0.65
Loyd Grossman Tikka Masala Curry Sauce	350	514.5	13.0	39.2	1.00
Sharwood's Tikka Masala Extra Creamy Curry Sauce	420	445.2	15.5	40.7	1.84
Sharwood's Tikka Masala Medium Curry Cooking Sauce	420	495.6	18.9	38.2	1.84

Values Shown Per Full Jar

Vindaloo Curry

Suggested Brands	Size (g)	Kcal	S.fat (g)	Carbs (g)	£
ASDA Vindaloo Curry	320	217.6	1.0	1.0	0.60
Morrisons The Best Goan Vindaloo Sauce	350	336.0	2.1	25.6	1.55
Patak's Vindaloo Curry	450	405.0	2.3	31.1	1.00
Indi Grand - Vindaloo Curry	375	487.5	30.0	37.5	0.60

Values Shown Per Full Jar

Soup

Soups are a great way of eating one of your five per day when using natural or organic vegetables in the recipe.

Thin soups are ideal when you need to satisfy hunger pangs very quickly. This type of soup also has the ability of exiting the body rapidly. This will allow the body to store the minimal number of calories, fats and sugars from the soup. This results in an improved digestive system, making you feel healthier and allows you to control your weight and health issues far easier.

Tomato soup will increase your resistance to cancer, soups containing celery will boost all the vitamins in the body. Chicken soup makes us feel better by moving around neutrophils (a type of blood cell) in the body when eaten. Historical claims of chicken soup having medical healing powers are a myth.

Chicken And Vegetable

Suggested Brands	Size (g)	Kcal	S.fat (g)	Carbs (g)	£
Heinz Eat Well Chicken, Vegetable & Quinoa	400	160.0	0.2	29.6	1.07
Baxters Favourites Chicken & Vegetable	400	164.0	0.4	25.2	1.07
Baxters Hearty Chicken & Vegetable	400	184.0	0.4	30.4	1.48
Slimming World Free Food	500	170.0	0.5	16.5	2.00
ASDA Chunky Chicken & Vegetable	400	180.0	0.8	17.2	0.63
Sainsbury's Chunky Chicken & Vegetable	400	184.0	0.8	22.0	0.60
Morrisons Chunky Chicken & Vegetable	400	184.0	0.8	19.2	0.75
Tesco Chunky Chicken And Vegetable	400	200.0	0.8	22.4	0.75
Heinz Chicken & Vegetable Big Soup	400	200.0	0.8	29.6	1.07
Crosse & Blackwell Best of British	400	164.0	2.4	20.0	1.07

Values Shown Per Full Can, Tub or Carton

Chicken Noodle

Suggested Brands	Size (g)	Kcal	S.fat (g)	Carbs (g)	£
Weight Watchers from Heinz	295	50.2	0.0	9.1	0.85
Heinz Chicken Noodle	400	128.0	0.4	24.4	0.95
Sainsbury's Asian Chicken	400	160.0	0.4	27.6	0.40
ASDA Classic	400	180.0	0.8	31.6	0.45
Sainsbury's Chicken	600	264.0	1.2	33.6	1.50
ASDA Chinese Chicken Noodle	600	1002.0	1.2	33.6	1.50
Baxters Super Good Chicken	400	200.0	1.6	26.4	1.00
Yorkshire Provender Thai Green	600	318.0	9.0	33.6	2.50

VALUES SHOWN PER FULL CAN, TUB OR CARTON

Chicken

Suggested Brands	Size (g)	Kcal	S.fat (g)	Carbs (g)	£
Weight Watchers Chicken Soup	295	91.5	0.3	13.3	0.85
Smart Price Chicken Soup	400	156	1.6	14	0.24
Heinz No Added Sugar Cream Of Chicken Soup	400	212	1.6	19.6	0.89
Heinz Cream Of Chicken	400	212	1.6	19.6	0.95
Tesco Everyday Value Chicken Soup	400	168.8	2	14.4	0.30
Tesco Cream Of Chicken Soup	400	193.6	2	11.2	0.45
Sainsbury's Cream Of Chicken Soup	400	216	2	20	0.40
ASDA Cream Of Chicken	400	216	2.4	19.2	0.39
Campbell's Condensed Cream Of Chicken	295	286.2	2.7	20.1	1.00
Essential Waitrose Cream Of Chicken Soup	400	276	3.6	19.6	0.52
Crosse & Blackwell Best Of British Roast Chicken	400	216	4	14	1.05
Baxters Favourites Cream Of Chicken Soup	400	232	4.8	23.2	1.10
New Covent Garden Classic Chicken	700	476	5.6	65.1	2.35

VALUES SHOWN PER FULL CAN, TUB OR CARTON

Leek And Potato

Suggested Brands	Size (g)	Kcal	S.fat (g)	Carbs (g)	£
ASDA Good & Balanced	500	275	0.0	52.5	1.00
Sainsburys	400	184	1.2	26.8	0.40
Baxter's Favourites Canned	400	208	1.2	28.8	1.07
ASDA Canned	400	164	2.0	28.0	0.45
Morrisons Canned	400	156	2.4	26.0	0.45
Tesco Canned	400	162	2.4	23.6	0.45
New Covent Garden Carton	600	330	3.6	29.4	2.00
Heinz Soup Of The Day	400	168	4.4	24.0	1.40
Heinz Canned	400	196	4.4	28.4	0.95
Crosse & Blackwell Best of British Canned	400	184	5.2	21.6	1.07
Waitrose (TUB)	600	276	6.0	33.0	1.99

Values Shown Per Full Can, Tub or Carton

Minestrone

Suggested Brands	Size (g)	Kcal	S.fat (g)	Carbs (g)	£
Heinz Minestrone	400	128.0	0.0	24.8	0.95
Slimming World Free Food Minestrone	500	180.0	0.0	29.5	2.00
ASDA Minestrone	400	148.0	0.2	25.2	0.45
Sainsbury's Minestrone	400	156.0	0.2	24.8	0.40
Baxters Vegetarian Minestrone	400	160.0	0.2	26.8	1.07
Morrisons Minestrone	400	136.0	0.4	22.8	0.45
Tesco Minestrone	400	160.0	0.4	28.8	0.45
Baxters Favourites Minestrone	400	168.0	0.8	28.0	1.07
Auga Organic	400	232.0	0.8	24.4	2.20

VALUES SHOWN PER FULL CAN, TUB OR CARTON

Mushroom

Suggested Brands	Size (g)	Kcal	S.fat (g)	Carbs (g)	£
Heinz Cream Of Mushroom	400	212	1.6	21.2	0.95
Tesco Cream Of Mushroom	400	240	2.04	23.12	0.45
ASDA Cream Of Mushroom	400	208	2.4	23.2	0.39
Sainsbury's Cream Of Mushroom	400	216	2.4	17.2	0.40
Campbell's Cream Of Mushroom	295	268.5	2.4	19.5	1.00
Essential Waitrose Cream Of Mushroom	400	240	4.8	16.8	0.52
Amy's Kitchen Organic Cream Of Mushroom	400	188	6	20	1.10
Baxters Favourites, Cream Of Mushroom	400	244	7.2	22	1.10
Cully And Sully Mushroom	400	264	12.8	9.2	1.50

VALUES SHOWN PER FULL CAN, TUB OR CARTON

Oxtail

Suggested Brands	Size (g)	Kcal	S.fat (g)	Carbs (g)	£
Heinz Oxtail	400	180.0	1.2	29.6	0.95
essential Waitrose oxtail	400	176.0	2.4	21.6	0.52
Morrisons Oxtail	400	172.0	2.8	21.6	0.45
ASDA Oxtail	400	176.0	2.8	20.8	0.39
Sainsbury's Oxtail	400	204.0	3.6	21.2	0.40

VALUES SHOWN PER FULL CAN, TUB OR CARTON

Pea And Ham

Suggested Brands	Size (g)	Kcal	S.fat (g)	Carbs (g)	£
ASDA Classic Pea & Ham	400	164.0	0.8	20.4	0.45
Morrisons Pea & Ham	400	164.0	0.8	20.4	0.45
Baxters Favourites Pea & Ham	400	200.0	0.8	26.4	1.07
Tesco Pea And Ham	400	212.0	0.8	27.6	0.45
Heinz Pea & Ham	400	256.0	0.8	38.4	0.95
Sainsbury's Pea & Ham	400	184.0	1.6	21.6	0.40
Crosse & Blackwell Best of British	400	284.0	4.0	32.8	1.05

VALUES SHOWN PER FULL CAN, TUB OR CARTON

Spicy Tomato

Suggested Brands	Size (g)	Kcal	S.fat (g)	Carbs (g)	£
ASDA Spicy Tomato	400	220.0	0.2	34.0	0.45
Sainsbury's Tomato & Spicy Lentil	400	232.0	0.2	37.6	0.40
Baxters Vegetarian Spicy Tomato & Rice	400	212.0	0.4	37.6	1.07
Heinz cream of tomato soup with fiery Mexican spice	400	244.0	0.8	28.4	1.35

VALUES SHOWN PER FULL CAN, TUB OR CARTON

Cream Of Tomato

Suggested Brands	Size (g)	Kcal	S.fat (g)	Carbs (g)	£
Smart Price Tomato	400	192	0.4	30	0.24
M savers Tomato	400	192	0.4	30	0.24
Heinz Cream of Tomato	400	204	0.8	27.2	0.95
Morrisons Cream of Tomato	400	212	0.8	24.8	0.45
essential Waitrose cream of tomato	400	212	0.8	24.8	0.52
Sainsbury's Cream Of Tomato	400	228	0.8	26.8	0.40
Tesco Cream Of Tomato	400	229.2	0.8	29.6	0.45
ASDA Cream of Tomato	400	232	0.8	29.2	0.39
Campbell's Condensed Cream of Tomato	295	137.8	0.9	19.8	1.00
Auga Organic Tomato Creamy	400	252	1.2	23.6	1.87
Amy's Kitchen Organic Chunky Tomato	400	204	3.2	34	1.60
Heinz Classic organic cream of tomato	400	224	3.6	28	1.29
Baxters Favourites Cream of Tomato	400	264	4	27.6	1.07

VALUES SHOWN PER FULL CAN, TUB OR CARTON

Vegetable

Suggested Brands	Size (g)	Kcal	S.fat (g)	Carbs (g)	£
Weight Watchers from Heinz Country	295	97.4	0.1	17.7	0.85
Sainsbury's Spring Vegetable	400	148.0	0.2	27.2	0.40
Morrisons Chunky Vegetable	400	148.0	0.2	24.4	0.75
ASDA Smart Price Vegetable	400	152.0	0.2	28.0	0.24
Sainsbury's Chunky Country	400	152.0	0.2	26.0	0.60
Morrisons Vegetable	400	168.0	0.2	25.2	0.45
ASDA Vegetable	400	180.0	0.2	32.8	0.45
Sainsbury's Vegetable	400	196.0	0.2	29.2	0.40
essential Waitrose	400	200.0	0.2	34.4	0.52
Heinz No Added Sugar Vegetable	400	168.0	0.4	28.8	0.89
Heinz Vegetable	400	188.0	0.4	33.2	0.95
Tesco Vegetable	400	200.0	0.4	32.4	0.45
Heinz Chunky Vegetable Big Soup	400	240.0	0.4	40.0	1.07
Baxters Hearty Country	400	192.0	1.2	30.0	1.00
Amy's Kitchen hearty rustic Italian	397	285.8	2.0	36.1	1.33
Amy's Kitchen Organic Hearty	400	360.0	2.0	44.0	1.80
Amy's Kitchen Hearty French Country	408	367.2	2.0	44.9	1.33
ASDA Classic Country Veg	400	180.0	3.2	25.6	0.45

SOUP   VEGETABLE

Suggested Brands	Size (g)	Kcal	S.fat (g)	Carbs (g)	£
Crosse & Blackwell Best of British Winter	400	256.0	4.0	38.4	1.07
Cully And Sully	400	248.0	10.4	18.0	1.50

VALUES SHOWN PER FULL CAN, TUB OR CARTON

Find Us On

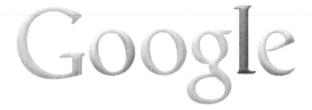

Search: **NADIET.INFO**

Canned Food

There is generally a good range of convenient canned food that you can heat very quickly using a saucepan or microwave. All canned food will show a list of ingredients with the calorie and nutritional information on the labelling so you know what you are eating. This is a better option compared to eating takeout or quick snacks, from food vendors, where you purchase processed convenience food where the calorie and nutritional information is generally unknown.

When reading calorie and nutritional information, always be aware that it is normal for the labelling on canned food to show as half can (or tin) as a food portion rather than the whole product. This easily catches people out where you think you are eating a product that contains 250 calories that is really 500 calories. This will negatively impact on your calorie counting and your desired lifestyle.

If you intend to eat canned food the following day, leave the can in the fridge overnight. All excess fat, nitrates and gelatin will travel to the top of the can when chilled. The following day keep the can upright and open, you can now scrape the excess fat, nitrates and gelatin from the top of the can using a small spoon. This is a great habit to form and will make the canned food tastier and healthier.

All Day Breakfast

Suggested Brands	Size (g)	Kcal	S.fat (g)	Carbs (g)	£
Hunger Breaks All Day Breakfast	395	418.7	4.7	44.2	1.25
Morrison's All Day Breakfast	395	446.4	5.1	47.8	1.27
Hunger Breaks The Full Monty	395	470.1	6.3	46.6	1.50

VALUES SHOWN PER FULL CAN

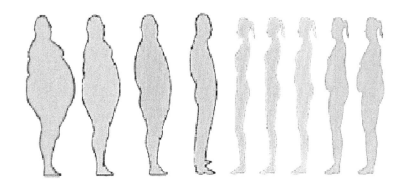

Baked Beans

Suggested Brands	Size (g)	Kcal	S.fat (g)	Carbs (g)	£
Weight Watchers	415	284	0	44.4	0.80
Heinz	415	323.7	0	51.9	0.75
Asda Reduced Sugar and Salt	410	299.3	0.4	40.6	0.31
Sainsbury's Basics	400	320	0.4	50.8	0.25
Smart price (Asda)	410	328	0.4	53.3	0.23
Sainsbury's	400	336	0.4	52	0.30
Essential Waitrose	400	348	0.4	54.8	0.32
Tesco Baked Beans	420	363.3	0.4	59.2	0.32
Asda home brand	410	373.1	0.4	61.5	0.30
Branston	410	348.5	0.8	56.6	0.65
Morrisons Baked Beans	410	369	0.8	56.6	0.32
Mr Organic	400	312	1.2	47.2	1.20
Tesco Everyday Value	405	460.4	5.7	51.6	0.41

VALUES SHOWN PER FULL CAN

Chilli Con Carne

Suggested Brands	Size (g)	Kcal	S.fat (g)	Carbs (g)	£
Tesco Everyday Value Chilli Con Carne	392	399.8	4.3	43.5	0.60
Smart Price Chilli Con Carne	392	392.0	4.7	28.2	0.55
Sainsbury's Chilli Con Carne, Basics	392	399.8	4.7	43.1	0.65
Tesco Chilli Con Carne	400	396.0	5.2	25.6	1.50
Tesco Hot Chilli Con Carne	400	420.0	5.6	24.8	1.50
Stagg Lite Reduced Fat Chili Con Carne Medium	400	440.0	6.4	52.0	1.79
Sainsbury's Chilli Con Carne	400	440.0	7.6	37.6	1.50
ASDA Chilli Con Carne	400	448.0	8.0	36.4	1.50
Stagg Classic Chili Con Carne	400	520.0	10.4	52.0	1.79
Stagg Chili Dynamite Hot Chili Con Carne	400	520.0	10.4	52.0	1.79
Princes Chilli Con Carne	392	576.2	15.7	35.7	1.79

VALUES SHOWN PER FULL CAN

Meat Balls

Suggested Brands	Size (g)	Kcal	S.fat (g)	Carbs (g)	£
Crosse & Blackwell 4Kids SBob in Gravy	370	310.8	2.6	33.3	0.78
Crosse And Blackwell 4Kids In Tomato Sauce	370	336.7	2.6	37.0	0.79
Smart Price in Tomato Sauce	380	357.2	2.7	33.4	0.48
Tesco In Tomato Sauce	395	377.6	4.3	43.6	0.60
Smart Price in Gravy	380	311.6	4.9	19.0	0.44
Morrisons In Gravy	380	357.2	5.3	31.2	0.67
Fray Bentos in Gravy	380	391.4	6.8	33.8	0.89
Fray Bentos in Onion Gravy	380	402.8	6.8	36.1	0.89
Fray Bentos in Tomato Sauce	380	437.0	6.8	43.3	0.89
Fray Bentos in Bolognese Sauce	380	440.8	6.8	44.5	0.89
Cooked Pork Meatballs in a Mexican Sauce	400	452.0	11.6	17.6	1.35
Can Cook Pork Meatballs in an Italian Sauce	400	460.0	23.2	39.2	1.35

VALUES SHOWN PER FULL CAN

Ravioli

Suggested Brands	Size (g)	Kcal	S.fat (g)	Carbs (g)	£
Sainsbury's Ravioli in Tomato Sauce	400	336	1.2	56	0.55
Smart price (Asda)	400	302	2.2	52	0.45
Asda home brand	400	324	2.6	50	0.55
Heinz	400	294	2.8	48	1.00
Tesco Beef Ravioli	400	324	3.2	52	0.55

VALUES SHOWN PER FULL CAN

Sausage Casserole

Suggested Brands	Size (g)	Kcal	S.fat (g)	Carbs (g)	£
ASDA Smart Price	390	315.9	4.7	31.6	0.98

VALUES SHOWN PER FULL CAN

Spaghetti In Tomato Sauce

Suggested Brands	Size (g)	Kcal	S.fat (g)	Carbs (g)	£
Heinz	400	240	0	50.4	0.75
Tesco Everyday Value	410	203.8	0.4	41	0.21
Sainsbury's Spaghetti Basics	400	204	0.4	40.4	0.20
Sainsbury's Spaghetti	400	204	0.4	39.6	0.30
Morrisons Spaghetti	395	233.1	0.4	47	0.35
Asda home brand	395	256.8	0.4	51.4	0.29
essential Waitrose short cut spaghetti	410	266	0.4	54.9	0.32
Tesco Short Cut Spaghetti	410	274.7	0.4	54.1	0.35
Smart price (Asda)	395	252.8	2.2	55.3	0.20

VALUES SHOWN PER FULL CAN

Spaghetti Bolognese

Suggested Brands	Size (g)	Kcal	S.fat (g)	Carbs (g)	£
Sainsbury's Vegetarian Spaghetti Bolognese	400	264.0	0.8	39.6	0.55
Heinz Spaghetti Bolognese	400	320.0	0.8	53.6	1.00
Branston Spaghetti Bolognese	395	272.6	1.6	40.7	1.00
Sainsbury's Spaghetti Bolognese	400	300.0	1.6	43.2	0.55
Tesco Everyday Value Spaghetti Bolognese	400	276.4	2.1	44.8	0.38
Morrisons Spaghetti Bolognese	395	288.4	2.4	39.1	0.64
ASDA Spaghetti Bolognese in Tomato Sauce	395	284.4	3.2	32.8	0.55
Sainsbury's Spaghetti Bolognese, Basics	400	448.0	3.2	63.2	1.00
Tesco Spaghetti Bolognese	400	340.8	5.9	34.4	0.55

VALUES SHOWN PER FULL CAN

Stewed Steak

Suggested Brands	Size (g)	Kcal	S.fat (g)	Carbs (g)	£
ASDA Stewed Steak	392	352.8	3.1	7.1	1.79
Grant's stewed steak	392	642.9	6.3	33.3	2.45
Sainsbury's Stewed Steak In Gravy	400	464.0	7.2	10.0	2.50
Morrisons Stewed Steak	392	458.6	7.4	12.5	2.00
Tesco Lean Stewed Steak	400	476.0	7.6	12.0	2.00
Princes Stewed Steak in a Rich Meaty Gravy	392	454.7	8.2	17.2	2.25
Stockwell & Co Stewed Steak & Gravy	400	468.0	9.6	17.6	1.59
ASDA Smart Price Stewed Steak	392	490.0	11.0	12.9	1.56

Values Shown Per Full Can

Korma Curry

Suggested Brands	Size (g)	Kcal	S.fat (g)	Carbs (g)	£
Sainsbury's Chicken Korma	400	596.0	21.2	11.2	1.50
ASDA Chicken Korma	400	696.0	25.6	19.2	1.00

Values Shown Per Full Can

Tomatoes

Suggested Brands	Size (g)	Kcal	S.fat (g)	Carbs (g)	£
Ktc Chopped	400	64	0	12	0.39
Smart Price Chopped	400	72	0	12	0.28
Smart Price Peeled Plum	400	72	0	12	0.28
Don Mario Chopped	400	72	0	12	0.50
Don Mario Plum	400	72	0	12	0.50
Tesco Everyday Value Plum	400	73.2	0	12	0.30
Ktc Plum Tomatoes	400	76	0	12	0.39
Napolina Chopped	400	92	0	14.4	1.05
Waitrose Cherry	395	98.4	0.0	15.0	0.82
Cook Italia Chopped	400	100	0	16	0.50
Napolina Chopped Tomatoes With Pepper & Chilli	400	100	0	16	0.75
Tesco Italian Chopped	400	100.8	0	16	0.35
Sainsbury's Italian Plum	400	80	0.04	14	0.40
Essential Waitrose Chopped	400	84	0.04	14.4	0.40
Waitrose Duchy Organic Chopped	400	88	0.04	14.8	0.89
Essential Waitrose Plum	400	92	0.04	15.2	0.40
Waitrose Duchy Organic Plum	400	92	0.04	13.6	0.84
Tesco Italian Finely Chopped	400	100.8	0.04	16	0.35
Tesco Peeled Plum	400	100.8	0.04	16	0.35
Morrison's Peeled Plum	400	104	0.04	20	0.40
Cirio Tinned Tuscan Plum	400	108	0.04	16.8	1.00

Suggested Brands	Size (g)	Kcal	S.fat (g)	Carbs (g)	£
Waitrose Chopped With Basil	400	112	0.04	19.6	0.65
Cirio Tinned Tuscan Chopped	400	116	0.04	18.8	1.00
Sainsbury's ChoppedSo Organic	400	80	0.4	11.2	0.80
Morrison's Italian Chopped	400	84	0.4	11.2	0.35
Sainsbury's Plum So Organic	400	84	0.4	12.4	0.80
Sainsbury's Peeled Plum Basics	400	88	0.4	16	0.30
Asda Italian Peeled Plum	400	88	0.4	15.2	0.35
Morrison's Chopped With Garlic & Onion	390	97.5	0.4	20.3	0.55
Asda Chopped	400	100	0.4	15.2	0.35
Sainsbury's Chopped Tomatoes With Basil	400	108	0.4	17.6	0.46
Waitrose Chopped With Olive Oil & Garlic	400	108	0.4	13.2	0.65
Sainsbury's Peeled Cherry	400	100	1.6	12.4	0.80

Values Shown Per Full Can

Tuna

Suggested Brands	Size (g)	Kcal	S.fat (g)	Carbs (g)	£
essential Waitrose Tuna Chunks in Spring Water	112	126.6	0.1	0.0	1.00
Skipjack Tuna Steaks in Brine	160	152.0	0.2	4.0	2.25
Princes Tuna Chunks In Spring Water	160	158.4	0.2	0.2	1.25
Sainsbury's Tuna Chunks Basics	160	180.8	0.2	0.5	0.80
Sainsbury's Tuna Chunks In Water	160	180.8	0.2	0.0	1.10
Sainsbury's Tuna in Brine	160	180.8	0.2	0.8	1.10
Princes Tuna Flakes in Brine	160	132.8	0.3	0.2	0.70
John West Tuna Chunks in Spring Water	145	163.9	0.3	0.0	0.88
Morrison's Tuna Chunks In Brine	160	174.4	0.3	0.0	0.93
Stockwell And Co Tuna Chunks In Brine	145	158.1	0.4	0.0	0.59
ASDA Smart Price Tuna Chunks in Brine	145	158.1	0.4	0.0	0.65
ASDA Skipjack Tuna Chunks in Spring Water	145	158.1	0.4	0.0	0.89
Tesco Tuna Chunks Brine	160	172.8	0.5	0.0	0.95
Tesco Tuna Chunks Spring Water	160	172.8	0.5	0.0	0.95
Essential Waitrose MSC tuna steak in spring water	150	177.0	0.6	0.0	1.50

Canned Food   Tuna

Suggested Brands	Size (g)	Kcal	S.fat (g)	Carbs (g)	£
Morrison's Tuna Chunks In Sunflower Oil	160	254.4	0.6	0.0	0.93
John West No Drain Tuna Steak with a Little Sunflower Oil	110	183.7	0.9	0.0	1.17
Skipjack Tuna Steaks in Organic Olive Oil	160	153.6	1.1	0.0	3.30
Sainsbury's Tuna Chunks In Olive Oil	160	302.4	2.4	0.8	1.15
Essential Waitrose MSC tuna steak in olive oil	150	313.5	3.0	0.0	1.50

Values Shown Per Full Can

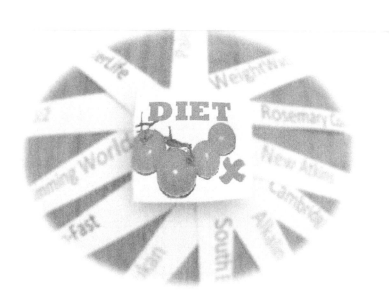

Readymade Meals

There is a good range of frozen convenient readymade food that you can heat very quickly using a conventional or microwave oven. All readymade food will show a list of ingredients with the calorie and nutritional information on the packaging so you know what you are eating. This is a better option compared to eating takeout or a quick snack, from food vendors, where you can purchase processed convenience food where the calorie and nutritional information is generally unknown.

If the packaging states the food has **reduced or lower** calories or fats, double check the nutritional information. Removing something from natural food normally means an alternative ingredient has replaced it. There is no legal requirement in 2020 for this alternative to be included on the ingredients list, so it could be anything. Best to avoid reduced or lower type foods if possible. Look for calorie counted, low in calorie or diet wording on the packaging instead.

Readymade meals can contain cheaper ingredients to maximise the financial profit for each of the food units sold. This less quality food will have a lower price and increased number of calories when compared to similar food brand. Why not try making your own pot meal at home, once ready you can split the food into serving sizes and freeze it creating your own readymade meals, and you know exactly the number of calories and the quality of the ingredients you have used.

All Day Breakfast

Suggested Brands	Size (g)	Kcal	S.fat (g)	Carbs (g)	£
Kershaws The All Day Big Breakfast	400	448	4.2	51.2	1.50
Hearty Food Co All Day	350	507.5	6.7	38.2	1.59
ASDA All Day Breakfast	350	528.5	6.7	42	1.50
Iceland All Day Breakfast	400	652	8.0	56.4	1.59
ASDA All Day Breakfast	400	620	8.8	52	2.20
Morrisons All Day Breakfast	400	804	13.2	52.4	3.00

VALUES SHOWN PER FULL MEAL

Beef Chilli And Rice

Suggested Brands	Size (g)	Kcal	S.fat (g)	Carbs (g)	£
Ilumi for Kids Disney Kitchen Beef Chilli & Rice	200	186.0	1.6	27.4	1.99
Kiddylicious Little Bistro Mild Beef Chilli With Rice	200	210.0	2.0	24.6	2.20
Morrisons Fresh Ideas One Pot Pulled Beef Chilli & Rice	360	414.0	2.2	53.6	3.26
LoveLife 3 Bean & Beef Chilli with Rice & Quinoa	370	473.6	4.1	63.6	3.99
Sainsbury's Beef Chilli With Coriander Rice	450	589.5	8.1	67.1	3.50

VALUES SHOWN PER FULL MEAL

Beef Dinner

Suggested Brands	Size (g)	Kcal	S.fat (g)	Carbs (g)	£
Sainsbury's Roast Beef Dinner	400	344.0	0.8	46.0	2.00
Tesco Roast Beef Dinner	400	340.0	1.2	43.2	1.75
Tesco Roast Beef Dinner 4+	400	428.0	1.2	53.2	3.70
Iceland Beef & Yorkshire Pudding Roast Dinner	450	414.0	1.8	51.8	1.59
Bisto Roast Beef Dinner	400	380.0	2.0	46.8	2.00
Morrisons Traditional Roast Beef Dinner	400	380.0	2.0	37.6	3.00
Waitrose Classic Roast Beef Dinner	390	417.3	2.3	50.3	4.50
ASDA Traditional Roast Beef Dinner	400	336.0	2.4	48.0	1.50

VALUES SHOWN PER FULL MEAL

Beef Lasagne

Suggested Brands	Size (g)	Kcal	S.fat (g)	Carbs (g)	£
ASDA Calorie Counted Beef Lasagne	380	364.8	2.7	49.4	2.40
Tesco Beef Lasagne	400	378.0	2.9	50.5	1.60
Weight Watchers from Heinz Beef Lasagne	320	288.0	3.5	35.2	1.75
ASDA Slimzone Beef Lasagne	500	435.0	3.5	36.0	2.00
Slimming World Free Food Beef Lasagne	550	561.0	4.4	58.9	3.50
Kirstys Classic Beef Lasagne	400	352.0	4.8	37.6	3.00
Morrisons Eat Smart Beef Lasagne	350	381.5	5.3	45.9	1.00
Sainsbury's Beef Lasagne, Be Good To Yourself	390	401.7	5.9	42.1	2.00
Morrisons Savers Beef Lasagne	400	404.0	6.0	40.0	1.00
ASDA Good & Counted Beef La	400	380.0	6.4	56.0	1.00
Bisto Beef Lasagne	375	412.5	7.1	49.5	1.25
Smart Price Beef Lasagne	400	336.0	7.2	32.4	1.00
Quorn Meat Free Classic Lasagne	500	545.0	7.5	65.5	3.20
Sainsbury's Deliciously Free From Beef Lasagne	400	536.0	7.6	58.8	2.50
Sainsbury's Beef Lasagne, Basics	400	484.0	8.4	55.2	1.00
Tesco Free From Beef Lasagne	430	593.4	9.0	71.4	3.00

READYMADE MEALS BEEF LASAGNE

Suggested Brands	Size (g)	Kcal	S.fat (g)	Carbs (g)	£
Sainsbury's Beef Lasagne	400	488.0	9.6	50.4	1.50
Waitrose beef lasagne	400	524.0	9.6	45.2	2.75
Sainsbury's Pub Specials Beef Lasagne	450	670.5	9.9	82.8	2.50
ASDA Beef Lasagne	400	476.0	10.0	52.0	0.88
ASDA Free From Beef Lasagne	350	458.5	10.5	49.0	2.75
Morrisons Beef Lasagne	400	512.0	10.8	49.2	1.00
Iceland Meal For One Beef Lasagne	500	670.0	11.5	64.0	1.00
ASDA Italian Beef Lasagne Al Forno	400	532.0	11.6	37.2	1.50
Tesco Beef And Pancetta Lasagne	400	538.8	12.6	46.7	2.00
ASDA Italian Beef Lasagne	450	621.0	12.6	45.0	2.20
Waitrose 1 Beef Lasagne	400	680.0	17.6	49.6	3.18
Iceland Luxury Beef & Pancetta Al Forno Lasagne	500	735.0	18.0	40.0	2.69
Waitrose 1 beef lasagne al forno	400	680.0	18.4	48.8	3.18
Tesco Beef Lasagne	450	652.5	18.5	45.9	2.50

VALUES SHOWN PER FULL MEAL

Chicken Chow Mein

Suggested Brands	Size (g)	Kcal	S.fat (g)	Carbs (g)	£
Tesco Slim Cook Chicken Chow Mein	500	310.0	0.5	38.0	2.50
Tesco Chicken Chow Mein 3+ days	400	260.0	0.8	32.8	2.50
Sainsbury's Chicken Chow Mein, Be Good To Yourself	400	300.0	0.8	31.2	3.00
Tesco Chicken Chow Mein	375	382.5	0.8	54.8	1.60
ASDA Slimzone Chicken Chow Mein	500	345.0	1.0	37.0	2.40
ASDA Takeaway Main Chicken Chow Mein	350	304.5	1.1	33.6	1.70
Iceland Chicken Chow Mein	375	401.3	1.1	50.6	1.59
Sainsbury's Chicken Chow Mein	400	324.0	1.2	41.2	1.60
Morrisons Chicken Chow Mein	400	344.0	1.2	44.4	1.65
ASDA Chicken Chow Mein	400	432.0	1.2	48.0	2.50
ASDA Chinese Chicken Chow Mein	400	336.0	1.6	40.0	1.50
Tesco Chicken Chow Mein	400	428.0	1.6	41.2	2.50
Sainsbury's Chicken Chow Mein	450	418.5	1.8	41.9	2.75
Waitrose chicken chow mein	400	432.0	2.0	50.8	3.69
Morrisons Oriental Chicken Chow Mein	400	492.0	2.0	61.2	2.50

VALUES SHOWN PER FULL MEAL

Chicken Curry And Rice

(Excluding Indian Flavours)

Suggested Brands	Size (g)	Kcal	S.fat (g)	Carbs (g)	£
Kershaws Chip Shop Chicken Curry with Rice & Chips	460	473.8	1.4	76.4	1.65
ASDA Smart Price Chicken Curry & Rice	400	300.0	2.8	36.4	1.10
Tesco Health Chicken Curry And Rice	350	322.0	2.8	50.1	1.20
ASDA Good & Counted Chinese Chicken Curry & Rice	350	322.0	3.2	52.5	1.05
Iceland Chinese Chicken Curry with Rice	400	588.0	3.6	69.2	1.65
ASDA Good & Balanced Chicken Katsu Curry and Rice	380	399.0	3.8	41.8	3.00
Morrisons Chicken Curry & Rice	400	524.0	6.0	82.8	1.00
Tesco Green Thai Chicken Curry & Rice	450	616.5	6.3	93.6	2.50
Tesco Finest Thai Green Chicken Curry & Coconut Jasmine Rice	410	508.4	7.4	60.3	3.50
Hearty Food Co. Chicken Curry With Rice	400	512.0	7.6	73.2	0.65
Iceland Chicken Curry with Rice	500	585.0	8.0	85.0	1.00

Readymade Meals Chicken Curry And Rice

Suggested Brands	Size (g)	Kcal	S.fat (g)	Carbs (g)	£
Tesco Finest Thai Red Chicken Curry & Coconut Jasmine Rice	440	646.8	9.2	76.6	3.50
Hungry Joe's Chicken Curry with Rice & Naan	600	768.0	9.6	114.0	2.20
Morrisons Thai Green Chicken Curry & Rice	400	524.0	10.0	66.0	1.80
ASDA Chicken Curry & Rice	400	592.0	10.0	72.0	0.90
Charlie Bigham's Thai Red Chicken Curry & Rice	418	606.1	18.8	56.8	4.85
Wasabi Sushi & Bento Thai Green Chicken Curry with Rice	450	621.0	20.3	63.5	4.00

Values Shown Per Full Meal

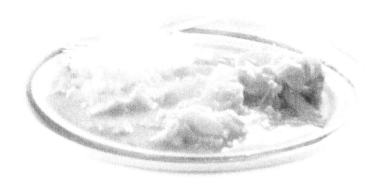

Chicken Dinner

Suggested Brands	Size (g)	Kcal	S.fat (g)	Carbs (g)	£
Kershaws Homestyle Chicken Dinner	400	272.0	0.8	40.4	1.73
Tesco Chicken Low Calorie Roast Dinner	400	288.0	0.8	28.8	2.50
Morrisons Counted Chicken Dinner	375	296.3	0.8	30.0	2.50
Morrisons Roast Chicken Dinner	400	396.0	0.8	50.8	3.00
M Counted Chicken Dinner	350	329.0	1.8	28.0	1.75
Tesco Classic Chicken Dinner	400	384.0	2.0	35.2	1.75
Morrisons Chicken Dinner	400	380.0	2.4	34.0	1.75
Tesco Chicken Roast Dinner	400	380.0	2.4	39.2	3.70
ASDA Roast Chicken Dinner	400	468.0	2.8	44.0	2.50
Iceland Chicken & Stuffing Roast Dinner	450	436.5	3.2	37.8	1.59
Birds Eye Traditional Chicken Dinner	400	376.0	3.6	40.0	2.50
Bisto Roast Chicken Dinner	400	456.0	3.6	41.2	2.50
Waitrose Classic Chicken Roast Dinner	420	558.6	4.6	51.7	4.50

VALUES SHOWN PER FULL MEAL

Chicken Korma and Rice

Suggested Brands	Size (g)	Kcal	S.fat (g)	Carbs (g)	£
Waitrose Lovelife Calorie Controlled Chicken Korma & Pilau Rice	400	420.0	2.0	64.4	3.50
Weight Watchers From Heinz Chicken Tikka Masala With Rice	310	334.8	2.5	49.0	1.25
Tesco Free From Chicken Korma And Rice	400	612.0	7.0	71.2	3.00
ASDA Indian Chicken Korma With Pilau Rice	400	624.0	8.4	84.0	1.50
Sainsbury's Indian Chicken Korma With Pilau Rice	450	742.5	8.6	89.6	3.00
Tesco Indian Chicken Korma And Rice	450	643.5	9.9	51.8	2.50
Sainsbury's Chicken Korma With Pilau Rice	400	684.0	10.4	83.2	1.50
ASDA Chicken Korma With Pilau Rice	450	778.5	11.3	85.5	2.20
Tesco Finest Chicken Korma And Rice	450	760.5	11.7	84.6	3.30
Iceland Meal For One Chicken Curry With Rice	500	630.0	13.0	87.0	1.00
Morrisons Indian Chicken Korma & Pilau Rice	450	742.5	13.1	85.5	2.40
Sainsbury's Fragrant Kashmiri Chicken Korma & Rice	450	805.5	14.0	81.5	4.00
Mumtaz Halal Chicken Korma & Rice	400	652.0	16.0	59.6	3.00

Suggested Brands	Size (g)	Kcal	S.fat (g)	Carbs (g)	£
Asda Extra Special Chicken Korma & Pilau Rice	400	732.0	16.0	64.0	3.50
Waitrose Chicken Korma & Pilau Rice	400	660.0	17.6	54.0	3.49
Charlie Bigham's Chicken Korma And Rice	405	688.5	21.1	59.5	4.00

VALUES SHOWN PER FULL MEAL

Please Remember to Subscribe for the Latest Updates

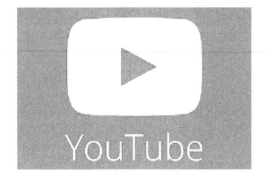

WWW.YOUTUBE.COM/STEPHENDBARNES

Classic Fish Pie

Suggested Brands	Size (g)	Kcal	S.fat (g)	Carbs (g)	£
Young's Low Fat Ocean Crumble	300	279.0	2.4	40.5	1.50
Young's Mariner's Pie	320	422.4	2.9	52.5	1.50
Young's Fisherman's Pie	320	371.2	4.2	44.2	1.20
Hearty Food Company Fish Pie	400	324.0	4.8	43.6	1.50
Tesco Fish Pie	400	324.0	4.8	45.7	2.50
ASDA Fish Pie	360	385.2	5.0	46.8	0.88
Waitrose Classic Fish Pie	400	384.0	6.0	38.8	2.75
Tesco Fish Pie	400	447.2	6.3	41.9	2.00
Young's Admiral's Pie	320	371.2	6.7	43.8	1.50
Morrisons Fishermans Pie	360	468.0	7.2	48.2	1.00
ASDA Extra Special Luxury Fish Pie	450	544.5	7.2	49.5	2.50
Smart Price Fish Pie	400	324.0	7.6	40.0	1.00
Young'S Gastro Our Fish Pie	400	472.0	8.0	41.6	2.20
Iceland Salmon Crumble	450	625.5	10.4	54.9	2.00
Sainsbury's Fish Pie, Taste the Difference	400	508.0	10.8	44.0	3.75
Sainsbury's Classic Cumberland Fish Pie	450	544.5	11.7	51.8	2.50
Waitrose 1 fish pie	400	488.0	12.0	36.8	3.18
Iceland Luxury Smoked Cod, Salmon & King Prawn Fish Pie	450	513.0	13.1	47.7	2.69
ASDA Classic Fish Pie	450	490.5	14.4	44.1	2.20

Suggested Brands	Size (g)	Kcal	S.fat (g)	Carbs (g)	£
Morrisons The Best Salmon Smoked Haddock & King Prawn Fish Pie	400	544.0	14.8	42.4	3.00
Tesco Finest Fish Pie	400	572.0	16.4	35.5	3.30
Charlie Bigham's Fish Pie	340	527.0	17.7	32.3	4.75

VALUES SHOWN PER FULL MEAL

Corn Beef Hash

Suggested Brands	Size (g)	Kcal	S.fat (g)	Carbs (g)	£
Home Made Corn Beef Hash (4 Servings)	400	332.1	5.0	25.9	0.95
ASDA Corned Beef Hash	450	522.0	5.0	54.0	2.20
Morrisons Corned Beef Hash	450	576.0	5.0	59.0	2.50
Waitrose Classic Corned Beef Hash	400	536.0	6.8	55.6	2.75
Tesco Corned Beef Hash	450	513.0	8.6	63.9	2.50
Iceland Classic Corned Beef Hash	450	688.5	11.3	61.2	2.00
Sainsbury's Classic Corned Beef Hash	450	625.5	14.4	38.3	2.00

VALUES SHOWN PER FULL MEAL

Cottage Pie

Suggested Brands	Size (g)	Kcal	S.fat (g)	Carbs (g)	£
Sainsbury's Lentil Cottage Pie	400	296.0	0.8	41.6	2.00
Asda Good & Counted	350	245.0	1.1	42.0	1.00
Waitrose Vegetable & Lentil Cottage Pie	380	410.4	1.1	49.4	2.80
Quorn Meat Free Cottage Pie	300	246.0	1.2	39.6	1.70
Morrisons Lentil Cottage Pie	400	296.0	1.6	40.8	2.50
Slimming World Free Food Cottage Pie	500	315.0	2.0	29.5	3.00
Kirstys Cottage Pie With Sweet Potato Mash	400	300.0	2.4	35.6	3.00
Morrisons Meat Free Cottage Pie	375	266.3	2.6	40.9	1.75
Weight Watchers From Heinz	320	252.8	2.9	30.4	1.39
Asda Calorie Counted	400	328.0	3.6	40.0	2.40
Waitrose Lovelife Calorie Controlled Cottage Pie	400	372.0	3.6	46.8	3.25
Sainsbury's Cottage Pie, Basics	300	282.0	4.2	36.9	1.00
Waitrose Frozen Vegetarian Cottage Pie	380	319.2	4.2	41.0	2.00
Bisto Cottage Pie	375	341.3	4.5	42.0	1.25
Asda Classic Cottage Pie	400	476.0	4.8	48.0	1.50
Hearty Food Co. Cottage Pie	400	352.0	5.2	40.8	1.20
Weight Watchers Hearty	400	328.0	5.6	36.0	2.50

READYMADE MEALS　COTTAGE PIE

Suggested Brands	Size (g)	Kcal	S.fat (g)	Carbs (g)	£
Morrisons The Best Cottage Pie With Real Ale Gravy	400	384.0	6.8	38.4	3.00
Tesco Classic Kitchen Cottage Pie	450	490.5	6.8	54.0	2.50
Asda Cottage Pie	400	440.0	7.2	44.0	0.88
Tesco Finest Cottage Pie	400	456.0	7.6	48.8	3.30
Sainsbury's British Classic Cottage Pie	450	414.0	7.7	41.9	2.00
Asda Vegetarian Carrot & Lentil	400	544.0	8.0	60.0	1.75
Morrisons Cottage Pie	400	420.0	8.8	39.2	1.00
Smart Price Cottage Pie	400	368.0	10.0	38.8	1.00
Asda Extra Special Cottage Pie	400	500.0	10.0	36.8	3.00
Waitrose Cottage Pie	400	460.0	11.2	27.2	2.75
Asda Cottage Pie	450	504.0	12.6	45.0	2.40
Waitrose Cottage Pie	400	580.0	13.2	41.2	3.18
Sainsbury's Cottage Pie, Taste The Difference	400	524.0	13.6	31.6	3.50
Charlie Bigham's Cottage Pie	325	552.5	14.6	30.2	5.00

VALUES SHOWN PER FULL MEAL

Macaroni Cheese

Suggested Brands	Size (g)	Kcal	S.fat (g)	Carbs (g)	£
Morrisons Macaroni Cheese	400	504.0	6.8	73.2	1.07
Sainsbury's Macaroni Cheese, Basics	300	429.0	8.4	50.1	1.00
Morrisons Savers Macaroni Cheese	400	480.0	8.8	68.8	1.00
Amy's Kitchen Gluten Free Rice Macaroni & Cheese	227	356.4	8.9	40.9	2.20
ASDA Macaroni Cheese	400	620.0	9.2	76.0	0.88
Iceland Meal For One Macaroni Cheese	500	650.0	9.5	90.0	1.00
Amy's Kitchen Gluten Free Rice Macaroni & Cheese	255	400.4	9.9	45.9	2.12
Iceland Luxury Crab Mac & Cheese	450	693.0	10.8	81.5	2.69
Smart Price Macaroni Cheese	400	492.0	11.6	60.0	1.00
Sainsbury's Love Your Veg! Macaroni Cheese & Jack Fruit	400	560.0	11.6	60.4	2.50
Hall's Macaroni Cheese with Ham Hock	400	1092.0	11.6	178.8	1.50
Iceland Luxury Beef Mac & Cheese	450	778.5	12.6	79.7	2.69
Sainsbury's Deliciously Free From Macaroni Cheese	400	544.0	12.8	83.2	3.00

Suggested Brands	Size (g)	Kcal	S.fat (g)	Carbs (g)	£
ASDA Free From Macaroni Cheese	400	772.0	14.8	108.0	2.40
Morrisons Mac & Cheese Bake	280	784.0	15.1	81.2	2.50
Tesco Macaroni Cheese	450	760.1	15.8	97.2	2.50
Waitrose Italian Macaroni Cheese with Cauliflower & Squash	400	752.0	16.0	81.2	2.75
ASDA Extra Special Pulled BBQ Beef Mac 'N' Cheese	400	820.0	16.0	80.0	3.50
ASDA Italian Macaroni Cheese	450	738.0	16.7	85.5	2.20
Waitrose Italian Macaroni Cheese with Bacon	400	828.0	17.2	86.0	2.75
Waitrose macaroni cheese	400	772.0	18.0	76.0	2.75
Sainsbury's Macaroni Cheese	400	672.0	18.8	67.6	2.00
ASDA Extra Special Four Cheese Macaroni	400	852.0	19.2	88.0	3.50
Sainsbury's Vintage Cheddar Mac & Cheese, Taste the Difference	375	738.8	20.6	70.5	3.50
Charlie Bigham's Macaroni Cheese	340	697.0	25.2	46.6	4.25

VALUES SHOWN PER FULL MEAL

Omelette

Suggested Brands	Size (g)	Kcal	S.fat (g)	Carbs (g)	£
Unearthed Spanish Omelette	200	316.0	3.0	24.0	1.85
Unearthed Spanish Spinach Omelette	300	402.0	3.6	29.7	2.99
Unearthed free range Spanish potato Omelette	300	465.0	5.4	28.2	2.49
Unearthed Spanish Omelette	500	710.0	7.5	47.5	3.59
Floristan Spanish Potato Omelette	500	765.0	8.0	65.0	2.50
Morrisons 2 Cheese Omelettes	200	426.0	10.2	5.6	1.00
Hearty Food Co. 2 Cheese Omelettes	200	452.0	11.0	8.2	0.65
ASDA 2 Cheese Omelettes	200	562.0	17.4	7.6	0.88

Values Shown Per Full Meal

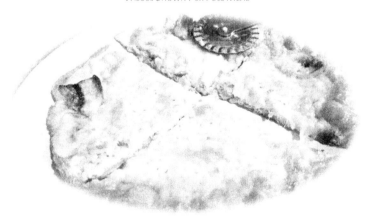

Pasta Bake

(Cheese, Tomatoes And Pasta)

Suggested Brands	Size (g)	Kcal	S.fat (g)	Carbs (g)	£
Morrisons Counted Tuna Pasta Bake	350	294.0	1.1	38.5	1.40
Morrisons Chicken Arrabiata & Tomato Pasta Bake	400	532.0	2.8	76.8	1.40
Hearty Food Co Cheese & Tomato Pasta	400	548.0	2.8	94.8	0.65
ASDA Cheese & Tomato Pasta Bake	400	504.0	3.2	84.0	0.90
Sainsbury's Tomato & Mozzarella Pasta	400	472.0	4.8	64.4	2.00
Tesco Tuna Pasta Bake	450	531.0	5.0	67.5	2.50
Tesco Tomato And Mozzarella Pasta Bake	450	535.5	5.9	76.5	2.50
Morrisons Italian Sausage Pasta Bake	400	648.0	6.0	82.4	2.50
Morrisons Italian Tuna Pasta Bake	400	524.0	6.4	56.0	2.50
Sainsbury's Chicken & Bacon Pasta	400	536.0	7.2	61.6	2.00
Waitrose Italian Tuna Pasta Bake	400	600.0	7.2	66.0	2.75
ASDA Smart Price Bolognese Pasta Bake	400	476.0	7.6	56.0	1.10
Sainsbury's Tuna Pasta Melt	400	488.0	7.6	56.4	2.00
Waitrose Italian Sausage Pasta Bake	400	608.0	8.0	81.6	2.75

Suggested Brands	Size (g)	Kcal	S.fat (g)	Carbs (g)	£
Tesco Pepperoni Pasta Bake	450	630.0	8.6	80.6	2.50
Tesco Pepperoni Pasta Bake	450	630.0	8.6	80.6	2.50
Tesco Chicken & Bacon Pasta Bake	450	657.0	10.4	67.5	2.50
Morrisons Italian Chicken & Bacon Pasta Bake	400	636.0	11.2	68.8	2.50
Sainsbury's Taste the Difference Chicken & Bacon Pasta Bake	375	611.3	13.1	49.9	3.00
Waitrose Italian Beef Bolognese Pasta Bake	400	716.0	13.6	72.0	2.75
Iceland Spicy Chilli Beef Pasta Bake	400	696.0	14.0	68.8	1.59
Morrisons Italian Meat Feast Pasta Bake	400	624.0	14.8	56.8	2.50

Values Shown Per Full Meal

Sausage And Mash

Suggested Brands	Size (g)	Kcal	S.fat (g)	Carbs (g)	£
Weight Watchers Lincolnshire Sausage & Root Vegetable Mash	380	292.6	3.0	32.7	2.50
Hearty Food Co Sausage And Mash	400	390.4	3.6	61.9	1.50
Tesco Sausage And Mash	400	340.0	3.8	43.9	2.50
Morrisons Eat Smart Counted Sausage & Mash	400	392.0	4.0	52.8	2.42
Hearty Food Company Sausages And Mash	400	404.0	4.0	53.6	1.20
ASDA Traditional Sausages & Mash	400	432.0	6.4	44.0	1.50
ASDA Filled Yorkshire Pudding with Sausages & Mash	430	731.0	6.5	90.3	2.40
Morrisons Savers Sausage & Mash	400	416.0	6.8	46.0	1.00
Waitrose Classics Sausage & Mash	430	481.6	7.3	50.7	2.75
Smart Price Sausage, Mash & Gravy	400	404.0	8.8	44.0	1.00
Tesco Bangers And Mash	450	508.5	9.7	54.0	2.50
ASDA Sausage & Mash	450	544.5	10.4	54.0	2.20
Iceland Meal For One Sausage & Mash	500	605.0	11.0	66.0	1.00
Iceland Classic Cumberland Sausage Ring & Mash	450	607.5	11.7	55.8	2.00

Readymade Meals Shepherd's Pie

Suggested Brands	Size (g)	Kcal	S.fat (g)	Carbs (g)	£
The Perfect Plate Sausage & Mash Dinner	420	571.2	13.4	41.2	2.69
ASDA Extra Special Cumberland Sausage & Mash	380	566.2	13.7	41.8	3.50
Tesco Finest Sausage And Mash	500	885.0	24.0	42.0	3.30

Values Shown Per Full Meal

Shepherd's Pie

Suggested Brands	Size (g)	Kcal	S.fat (g)	Carbs (g)	£
Tesco Shepherd's Pie	450	378.0	4.5	53.1	2.50
Bisto Shepherd's Pie	375	322.5	5.3	35.6	1.25
Asda Shepherd's Pie	400	344.0	6.0	40.0	0.88
Hearty Food Company Co. Shepherd's Pie	400	324.0	7.1	29.6	1.00
Tesco Finest Shepherd's Pie	400	436.0	7.7	48.3	3.30
Sainsbury's Shepherd's Pie	400	392.0	8.4	38.8	1.50
Morrisons Shepherd's Pie	450	450.0	9.5	48.2	2.23
Waitrose Shepherd's Pie	400	440.0	10.0	43.2	2.75
Morrisons The Best Shepherd's Pie	400	508.0	10.4	51.6	3.00
Morrisons Shepherd's Pie	400	472.0	11.2	39.6	1.57

Values Shown Per Full Meal

Sliced Beef In Gravy

Suggested Brands	Size (g)	Kcal	S.fat (g)	Carbs (g)	£
Hearty Food Co. Sliced Beef In Gravy	210	117.6	0.2	8.0	0.65
Bisto Best Beef & Red Wine Rich Gravy Sauce	150	76.5	0.3	9.0	1.49
ASDA Beef in Gravy	210	134.4	1.3	10.1	0.90
Iceland Sliced Beef in Gravy	200	142.0	1.6	9.8	1.00
Morrisons Beef Slices In Gravy	210	268.8	2.9	12.6	1.10
ASDA Slow Cooked Beef Brisket in Stout Gravy	300	450.0	6.9	8.1	3.25
Tesco Beef Brisket In Gravy	400	608.0	12.8	12.4	3.50

VALUES SHOWN PER FULL MEAL

Spaghetti Bolognese

Suggested Brands	Size (g)	Kcal	S.fat (g)	Carbs (g)	£
Morrisons Savers Spaghetti Bolognese	400	332.0	1.6	53.6	1.00
Morrisons Eat Smart Counted Spaghetti Bolognese	400	320.0	2.0	44.0	2.42
Sainsbury's Spaghetti Bolognese, Basics	300	276.0	2.4	38.7	1.00
ASDA Calorie Counted Spaghetti Bolognese	380	376.2	2.7	49.4	2.40
Iceland Meal For One Spaghetti Bolognese	500	540.0	3.0	82.0	1.00
Bisto Spaghetti Bolognese	375	337.5	3.4	45.8	1.25
Morrisons Italian Spaghetti Bolognese	400	436.0	5.6	51.6	2.23
Morrisons Spaghetti Bolognese	400	472.0	5.6	62.0	1.00
ASDA Spaghetti Bolognese	400	504.0	6.0	68.0	0.88
ASDA Italian Spaghetti Bolognese	450	603.0	6.8	72.0	2.20
Sainsbury's Spaghetti Bolognese	400	468.0	7.6	48.8	2.00
Waitrose spaghetti Bolognese	400	560.0	7.6	76.4	2.75
ASDA Free From Spaghetti Bolognese	400	576.0	9.2	64.0	2.40
Sainsbury's Deliciously Free From Spaghetti Bolognese	400	604.0	9.2	70.8	3.00

READYMADE MEALS   SPAGHETTI BOLOGNESE

Suggested Brands	Size (g)	Kcal	S.fat (g)	Carbs (g)	£
Sainsbury's Slow Cooked Spaghetti Bolognese, Taste the Difference	400	592.0	11.2	43.2	3.50
Iceland Italian Spaghetti Bolognese	400	612.0	11.6	50.8	1.59
ASDA Extra Special West Country Beef	450	688.5	12.6	54.0	3.50

VALUES SHOWN PER FULL MEAL

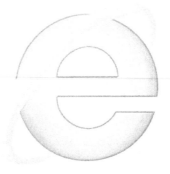

Find Us on The Web

WWW.WECANTSPELLSUCCESSWITHOUTYOU.COM

&

WWW.NADIET.INFO

Sweet And Sour Chicken With Rice

Suggested Brands	Size (g)	Kcal	S.fat (g)	Carbs (g)	£
Weight Watchers Sweet & Sour Chicken	320	380.8	0.6	70.4	1.75
Morrisons Counted Sweet & Sour Chicken With Rice	350	413.0	0.7	71.4	1.00
Tesco Sweet & Sour Chicken With Egg Fried Rice	380	380.0	0.8	58.9	2.50
Sainsbury's Sweet & Sour Chicken & Rice, Be Good To Yourself	380	391.4	0.8	56.6	3.00
ASDA Sweet & Sour Chicken With Rice	400	448.0	0.8	76.0	0.90
Hearty Food Company Sweet & Sour Chicken With Rice	400	460.0	0.8	78.4	1.10
Iceland Sweet & Sour Chicken with Egg Fried Rice	400	572.0	0.8	91.2	1.65
Hearty Food Company Sweet & Sour Chicken With Rice	400	448.0	1.2	86.0	0.65
Iceland Sweet & Sour Chicken with Rice	500	685.0	2.0	119.0	1.00
Morrisons Sweet & Sour Chicken with Egg Fried Rice	450	621.0	2.3	87.3	2.50
Sainsbury's Crispy Sweet & Sour Chicken With Rice	400	712.0	2.4	94.0	3.00

Suggested Brands	Size (g)	Kcal	S.fat (g)	Carbs (g)	£
Sainsbury's Sweet & Sour Chicken With Rice	450	715.5	2.7	101.7	2.75
ASDA Chinese Sweet & Sour Chicken with Egg Fried Rice	400	492.0	2.8	80.0	1.50
Tesco Sweet & Sour Chicken Egg Fried Rice	400	544.0	2.8	85.6	1.60
Sainsbury's Sweet & Sour Chicken With Rice	400	612.0	4.4	83.6	1.60
Tesco Sweet & Sour Chicken & Rice	450	751.5	5.4	92.3	2.50

VALUES SHOWN PER FULL MEAL

Tikka Masala With Pilau Rice

Suggested Brands	Size (g)	Kcal	S.fat (g)	Carbs (g)	£
Tesco Healthy Living Chicken Tikka Masala & Pilau Rice	400	408.0	2.0	59.2	2.50
Waitrose LoveLife Calorie Controlled chicken tikka masala with pilau rice	400	444.0	2.0	63.6	3.50
Iceland Chicken Tikka Masala with Pilau Rice	400	608.0	2.0	94.0	1.65
ASDA Prawn Tikka Masala with Pilau Rice	400	516.0	3.2	84.0	1.65
Patak's Chicken Tikka Masala with Pilau Rice	400	584.0	3.6	70.8	1.75
ASDA Indian Chicken Tikka Masala with Pilau Rice	400	596.0	4.0	88.0	1.50
Tesco Vegetable Tikka Masala With Rice	450	508.5	5.9	68.9	2.50
Tesco Chicken Tikka Masala Pilau Rice	400	512.0	6.0	52.4	1.60
ASDA Chicken Tikka Masala with Pilau Rice	400	596.0	6.0	72.0	2.10
Sainsbury's Indian Chicken Tikka Masala with Pilau Rice	400	560.0	6.4	61.6	2.25
Morrisons Indian Hot Chicken Tikka Masala & Pilau Rice	450	576.0	8.1	52.7	2.50
Morrisons Indian Chicken Tikka Masala & Pilau Rice	450	675.0	9.5	73.4	2.50

Suggested Brands	Size (g)	Kcal	S.fat (g)	Carbs (g)	£
Waitrose chicken tikka masala with pilau rice	400	624.0	11.2	53.6	3.50
ASDA Extra Special Chicken Tikka Masala & Pilau Rice	400	636.0	11.6	60.0	3.50
Charlie Bigham's Chicken Tikka Masala & Pilau Rice for 1	403	737.5	24.2	61.7	4.85

VALUES SHOWN PER FULL MEAL

Toad In The Hole

Suggested Brands	Size (g)	Kcal	S.fat (g)	Carbs (g)	£
Aunt Bessie's Vegetarian Toad In The Hole	190	313.5	1.3	26.6	1.85
Quorn Meat Free	200	384.0	1.6	39.4	1.70
Morrisons Toad In The Hole 3	300	489.0	4.5	60.9	1.00
Aunt Bessie's Toad In The Hole	190	345.8	4.6	30.4	1.00
Iceland Toad in the Hole	300	513.0	6.0	55.8	1.00
Bisto Toad In The Hole	300	603.0	6.6	69.6	1.00
ASDA Toad in the Hole	300	552.0	7.2	57.0	0.90
Hearty Food Co. Toad In The Hole	300	624.0	7.2	69.9	0.65
ASDA Toad in the Hole	340	924.8	18.7	64.6	2.30
Tesco Toad In The Hole	340	911.2	19.7	64.6	2.50
The Real Yorkshire Pudding Co. Toad in the Hole	350	1032.5	23.1	80.5	2.50

Values Shown Per Full Meal

Notes

Snacks

Snacks can be high in calories so avoid using them late at night as this will allow carbohydrate and sugar to easily convert to fat. If you love to snack at night, choose a low sugar food or even better eat fruit, veg or pickled onions. All of these will contain natural sugars that the body will find harder to convert to fat.

Historically, we would have elevenses where we would drink tea or coffee and enjoy a nice cake or scone. This is the time to eat our favourite cake or sugary snack, as we will remain active during the day while achieving your step challenge. This allows the sugar from the snack to convert to energy rather than being stored as fat in the body.

If you are looking at weight gain, late night snacking is the answer. Always choose a low carbohydrate option to avoid becoming at risk of diabetes type 2. These lower carbohydrate options will allow you to eat more of your favourite snack safely without the risk of damaging your health.

Black Peas

Suggested Brands	Size (g)	Kcal	S.fat (g)	Carbs (g)	£
Baxter's Hearty Chicken Black Eyed Peas	400	184	0.4	26.8	1.47

VALUES SHOWN PER PRODUCT

Cheese And Onion Pie or Bakes

Suggested Brands	Size (g)	Kcal	S.fat (g)	Carbs (g)	£
Morrisons 2 Cheese & Onion Bakes	280	282	2.7	31.9	1.50
Holland's 4 Cheese & Onion Pies	740	443	9.2	50	2.00
ASDA 2 Cheese & Onion Bakes	280	359	10	35	1.00
Linda McCartney Cheese Leek & Red Onion Plaits (2)	340	456	14.8	38.6	1.83
Greggs 2 Cheese & Onion Bakes	288	434	16	33	1.00
Higgidy Oak Smoked Cheddar & Onion Pie	200	602	17	48.8	3.10

VALUES SHOWN PER PIE

Chocolate Bars

Suggested Brands	Size (g)	Kcal	S.fat (g)	Carbs (g)	£
Alpen Light Chocolate & Fudge Bars	19	65.0	0.5	10.5	1.50
Milky Way Chocolate Bar 6x21.5g	21.5	96.8	1.7	15.2	1.50
Cadbury Fudge Chocolate Bar 6x25.5	25.5	113.5	2.1	19.0	1.25
Milkybar White Chocolate Bar 6 Pack	12	65.2	2.3	6.4	1.00
Cadbury Snack Shortcake Chocolate Biscuit 6 Pack	20	96.6	2.4	11.4	1.00
Blue Riband Original Milk Chocolate Wafer	18	92.3	2.5	11.8	1.00
Cadbury Curly Wurly Chocolate Bar	26	117.8	2.5	18.2	1.25
Cadbury Time Out Wafer Chocolate	16	84.3	2.6	9.6	1.00
Breakaway Milk Chocolate Biscuit Bar 8 Pack	19	97.1	2.6	12.1	1.00
Fox's Rocky Caramel 8 Bars	21	98.3	2.7	13.4	0.85
Cadbury Crunchie Chocolate Bar 4 Pack	32	149.1	3.2	23.4	1.00
Mars Chocolate Bar	39.4	176.5	3.2	27.3	2.50
Cadbury Dairy Milk Freddo Chocolate Bar 6x18g	18	95.4	3.3	10.2	1.25
Yorkie Milk Chocolate Biscuit Bar 7 Pack	24.5	123.7	3.3	15.3	1.00

SNACKS CHOCOLATE BARS

Suggested Brands	Size (g)	Kcal	S.fat (g)	Carbs (g)	£
Topic Chocolate Bar 4x47	47	229.4	3.7	29.0	1.50
McVitie's Penguin Original Chocolate Biscuit Bar 8 Pack	24.6	128.2	3.8	15.4	1.00
Cadbury Twirl Chocolate Bar	21.5	115.0	3.9	12.3	2.50
McVitie's Club Orange Bars	24	122.9	4.0	14.6	1.00
Snickers Chocolate Bar	41.7	212.7	4.0	22.7	1.50
Snickers Chocolate Bar	41.7	212.7	4.0	22.7	2.50
Bahlsen PiCK UP! Milk Chocolate Biscuit Bars	28	143.1	4.2	17.1	1.00
McVitie's Trio Toffee Biscuit Bar 6 Pack	23	121.2	4.4	13.6	1.00
Lion Peanut Chocolate Bar 4 Pack	41	202.5	4.4	22.5	1.00
Cadbury Double Decker Chocolate Bar 4 Pack	47	217.6	4.4	33.8	1.00
Aero Mint Bubbly Chocolate Bar 4 Pack	27	143.4	4.6	16.6	1.00
Cadbury Flake Chocolate Bar 4 Pack	25.5	136.4	4.8	14.3	1.00
McVitie's Gold Bar	24	124.3	5.0	16.0	1.00
KitKat Chunky Chocolate Bar	40	202.8	5.6	25.0	1.00
Galaxy Ripple Chocolate Bar	33	174.6	5.7	19.4	1.50
Cadbury Wispa Chocolate Bar 4 Pack	30	165.0	6.3	15.8	1.00
Toffee Crisp Chocolate Bar	38	198.0	6.7	23.9	1.00

Suggested Brands	Size (g)	Kcal	S.fat (g)	Carbs (g)	£
Twix Chocolate Bar	50	247.0	6.9	32.3	2.50
Kinder Bueno Milk and Hazelnuts Chocolate Bar 4 Pack	43	246.0	7.4	21.3	2.00
Tesco Free From Chocolate Bar	35	190.4	7.6	16.9	0.45
Eat Natural Bar, Cranberry Macadamia & Chocolate Gluten Free	45	214.7	8.0	15.9	2.00
Galaxy Milk Chocolate Bar 4x42g	42	229.3	8.2	23.5	1.50
Bounty Chocolate Bar 4	57	278.2	12.2	33.3	1.50
Lindt Excellence Chocolate Bar Dark Orange Intense	100	526.0	18.0	49.0	2.00
Lindt Excellence Chocolate Bar Dark Mint Intense	100	529.0	19.0	51.0	2.00
Cadbury Dairy Milk Whole Nut Chocolate Bar	120	660.0	19.8	58.8	1.50
Green & Black's Organic Milk Chocolate Bar	100	561.0	22.0	48.0	1.50
Green & Black's Organic 70% Dark Chocolate Bar	90	522.0	22.5	32.4	2.00
Lindt Excellence Chocolate Bar Dark	100	566.0	24.0	34.0	2.00
Green & Black's Organic 85% Dark Chocolate Bar	90	546.3	27.0	21.6	2.00
Tesco Intense Dark Chocolate Bar	100	585.0	29.0	22.0	1.00

SNACKS CHOCOLATE BARS

Suggested Brands	Size (g)	Kcal	S.fat (g)	Carbs (g)	£
Lindt Excellence Chocolate Bar Dark 90% Cocoa	100	592.0	30.0	34.0	2.00
Cadbury Dairy Milk Caramel Chocolate Bar	200	980.0	30.0	119.0	2.00
Cadbury Dairy Milk Chocolate Bar	200	1068.0	36.0	114.0	2.00
ASDA Milk Chocolate Bar	200	1078.0	38.0	116.0	0.90
Tesco Dark Chocolate Bar	200	1064.0	40.0	98.0	1.00
Tesco White Chocolate Bar	200	1166.0	48.0	106.0	1.00

VALUES SHOWN PER CHOCOLATE BAR

Chocolate Cakes

Suggested Brands	Size (g)	Kcal	S.fat (g)	Carbs (g)	£
Sainsbury's Chocolate Fairy Cakes (12)	12	85.0	0.5	9.6	1.00
ASDA Chocolate Fairy Cakes (12)	12	89.0	0.5	10.0	0.85
Sainsbury's Chocolate & Vanilla Marble Loaf Cake (6)	200	133.3	1.0	17.5	1.60
ASDA Baker's Selection 20 Chocolate Cluster Mini Bites	20	47.0	1.1	7.0	2.00
Morrisons Chocolate Cake Slices (6)	6	126.0	1.1	15.2	1.00
ASDA Chocolate Brownie Traybake (6)	225	155.6	1.1	21.8	1.00
ASDA Mini Chocolate Cupcakes (9)	9	108.0	1.5	12.0	2.00
ASDA Chocolate Sponge (6)	6	123.0	1.5	21.0	1.00
Weight Watchers Chocolate Mini Rolls(5)	5	80.0	1.6	12.8	1.30
Mr Kipling Chocolate Slices(8)	8	132.0	1.9	18.0	2.25
Sainsbury's Chocolate Party Cake (12)	930	300.7	2.0	41.5	6.00
Sainsbury's Deliciously Free From Seriously Chocolate Cake (10)	612	265.6	2.1	36.8	8.00
Tunnock's Milk Chocolate Tea Cakes (6)	6	106.0	2.5	14.9	1.05

SNACKS CHOCOLATE CAKES

Suggested Brands	Size (g)	Kcal	S.fat (g)	Carbs (g)	£
Cadbury 5 Milk Chocolate Cake Bars (5)	5	110.0	2.7	13.3	1.60
ASDA White Chocolate & Raspberry Celebration Cake (28)	1000	165.0	2.9	21.8	10.00
ASDA 4 Chocolate Eclairs (4)	4	101.0	3.0	8.4	1.00
Cadbury Chocolate Mini Rolls (5)	5	115.0	3.1	13.6	1.50
Thorntons Triple Chocolate Cake Bites (9)	9	62.0	3.2	7.7	1.50
McVitie's 5 Caramel Millionaire Slices with Milk Chocolate	5	116.0	3.4	13.9	0.75
ASDA Free From Chocolate Loaf Cake (5)	330	267.3	3.4	37.6	3.00
ASDA Free From Chocolate Party Cake (10)	656	268.3	3.5	32.8	7.00
Cadbury Flake Chocolate Fresh Cream Cake (8)	430	173.6	3.6	21.4	3.50
Just Love Food Company Let's Celebrate! Celebration Cake (10)	579	228.1	3.9	27.4	6.00
Sainsbury's Chocolate Chip Slab Cake (10)	500	193.0	4.0	28.2	1.40
Tesco Hot Chocolate Fudge Cake (6)	450	255.8	4.0	21.7	1.50
Iceland Celebration Chocolate Cake (16)	950	245.2	4.3	32.8	5.00
Thorntons Chocolate Celebration Cake (18)	990	240.9	4.5	27.0	12.00

Suggested Brands	Size (g)	Kcal	S.fat (g)	Carbs (g)	£
Baileys Chocolate Cupcakes With Buttercream Topping (12)	12	230.0	4.6	28.1	8.00
Sainsbury's Belgian Chocolate Fudge Cake, Taste Difference (6)	395	281.8	4.6	34.6	2.00
Sainsbury's Small Seriously Chocolate Cake (10)	550	241.5	4.9	29.2	6.50
Sainsbury's Seriously White Chocolate Madeira Cake (12)	839	304.1	5.1	41.7	10.00
ASDA Chocolate Gateau (5)	350	183.4	5.3	21.7	1.35
Sainsbury's Chocolate Sweetie Smash Cake (16)	913	265.9	5.4	31.0	13.00
Waitrose Chocolate Sweetie Cake (14)	800	254.3	5.5	30.5	12.00
Mary Berry Indulgent Chocolate Cake (6)	420	292.6	5.6	36.9	3.50
Tesco Hot Chocolate Fudge Cake (8)	700	274.8	5.9	38.5	5.50
Waitrose Hand Finished Chocolate Cake (12)	760	276.1	6.0	31.5	8.00
Iceland Chocolate Fudge Cake (6)	450	261.0	6.1	32.8	1.50
Morrisons Chocolate Fudge Frozen Cake (6)	450	267	6.1	33.8	1.60
ASDA Chocolate Cake Slice (1)	100	398.0	6.1	52.0	1.09

Suggested Brands	Size (g)	Kcal	S.fat (g)	Carbs (g)	£
Waitrose White Chocolate Cake (12)	885	330.4	6.3	43.7	10.00
Galaxy Chocolate Mousse Cake (6)	425	250.8	8.5	23.4	2.00
Waitrose 1 chocolate & salted caramel mini cakes (2)	2	308.0	8.5	38.9	2.49
Almondy Daim Chocolate Cake (2)	400	848.0	18.0	88.0	3.00

VALUES SHOWN PER SLICE OR INDIVIDUAL CAKE

Crisps

Suggested Brands	Size (g)	Kcal	S.fat (g)	Carbs (g)	£
Skips	17	92	0.5	9.9	0.55
Tesco everyday salt and vinegar *	18	98	0.5	9.2	0.05
Walkers Quavers	20	107	0.5	12.0	0.55
Tesco everyday Cheese And Onion *	18	95	0.6	9.6	0.05
Tesco everyday Ready Salted *	18	96	0.6	9.5	0.05
Smart Price Ready Salted *	18	99	0.6	9.3	0.05
Walkers Smoky Bacon	25	130	0.6	13.4	0.45
Tesco Smoky Bacon *	25	87	0.7	12.6	0.13
Asda Ready Salted *	25	130	0.7	13	0.13
Asda Roast Chicken	25	130	0.7	13	0.13
Asda Cheese And Onion *	25	132	0.7	13	0.13
Morrison's smoky bacon *	25	132	0.7	13.8	0.13
Tesco salt and vinegar *	25	134	0.7	13	0.08
Tesco Roast Chicken *	25	134	0.7	12.3	0.13
Morrison's Roast chicken *	25	134	0.7	12.3	0.13
Tesco Cheese And Onion *	25	134	0.7	13	0.13
Tesco Prawn Cocktail *	25	135	0.7	12.7	0.08
Tesco Ready Salted *	25	136	0.7	13.8	0.08
Asda salt and vinegar *	25	132	0.8	13	0.13
Asda Prawn Cocktail *	25	133	0.8	13	0.13
Morrison's everyday Ready Salted *	25	136	0.8	13.1	0.13
Walkers Roast Chicken	32.5	168	0.8	17.1	0.55

Suggested Brands	Size (g)	Kcal	S.fat (g)	Carbs (g)	£
Walkers Cheese And Onion	32.5	169	0.8	17.1	0.55
Walkers salt and vinegar	32.5	169	0.8	17.1	0.55
Walkers Prawn Cocktail	32.5	169	0.8	17.2	0.55
Walkers Ready Salted	32.5	171	0.8	16.7	0.55

VALUES SHOWN PER PACKET

* INDICATES SOLD AS MULTIPACK, PRICE SHOWN IS PER MULTIPACK

Meat And Potato Pie

Suggested Brands	Size (g)	Kcal	S.fat (g)	Carbs (g)	£
Holland's 4 Meat & Potato	Per Pie	385	6.6	42	2.00
Greggs 2 Meat and Potato Pies	Per Pie	769.6	13.5	72.5	2.50
Dicksons Corned Beef and Potato Family Plate Pie	¼ Pie	481.8	14.6	28.3	3.49

VALUES SHOWN PER PIE

Pasties / Slice

Suggested Brands	Size (g)	Kcal	S.fat (g)	Carbs (g)	£
TS Foods Tony's Chippy 4 Pasties	400	267.0	2.9	27.0	1.75
Ginsters Original Cornish Pasty (5 pack)	227	114.0	3.2	9.6	1.50
Quorn 2 Pasties	300	319.5	7.5	33.8	2.00
Peter's Chicken Pasty	150	396.0	7.8	39.8	0.95
ASDA 2 Chicken Tikka Slices	300	370.5	8.1	36.0	1.75
2 Beef Pasties	300	354.0	8.7	36.5	1.15
Tesco 2 Pulled Pork Slices	300	372.0	8.9	38.1	1.75
Eastmans Chicken And Mushroom Slice	150	337.5	9.2	32.3	0.52
ASDA 2 Chicken & Bacon Slices	300	399.0	9.5	36.0	1.75
Wicked Kitchen Curried Cauliflower Pasty	150	361.5	9.8	39.3	1.60
Dicksons Corned Beef & Potato Twin Pack Pasty	280	389.2	10.0	36.1	1.89
ASDA Smart Price Minced Beef & Vegetable Pasty	150	385.5	10.1	37.5	0.39
ASDA 2 Steak Slices	300	405.0	10.2	39.0	1.75
ASDA 5 Cornish Pasties	675	363.2	10.3	29.7	2.27
Ginsters 2 Westcountry Cheddar & Onion Pasties	260	338.0	10.4	28.9	1.60
ASDA Cheese & Onion Pasty	150	402.0	10.4	43.5	0.39
Tesco 4 Cheese And Onion Pasties 520G	520	351.0	10.9	28.5	1.75
Peter's Corned Beef Pasty	150	379.5	11.0	64.8	0.95

Suggested Brands	Size (g)	Kcal	S.fat (g)	Carbs (g)	£
Ginsters Moroccan Vegetable Pasty	180	408.6	11.0	42.5	1.50
Tesco Cornish Pasty	130	370.5	11.6	26.1	0.75
Tesco 4 Cornish Pasties	520	370.5	11.6	26.1	1.75
Morrisons Cornish Pasties x 4	520	373.1	11.7	25.9	1.75
Eastmans Minced Beef And Onion Pasty	150	430.5	11.9	38.3	0.39
Peter's Traditional Pasty	199	511.4	11.9	51.1	0.95
Sainsbury's Cornish Pasties x4	600	415.5	12.0	34.1	2.10
ASDA 2 Sausage & Cheesy Bean Slices	300	468.0	12.0	45.0	1.75
The Welsh Pantry Monster Bite Minced Beef & Vegetable Pasty	300	366.0	12.2	38.4	1.15
Tesco Counter Beef And Vegetable Pasty	150	466.5	12.3	40.1	2.00
Ginsters Chicken & Mushroom Slice	170	431.8	12.6	33.8	1.60
Fry's Vegan Spicy 3 Bean Pasty	200	498.0	12.8	53.4	1.30
Morrisons Cheese & Onion Pasties x 4	520	404.3	13.0	28.6	1.75
Ginsters Peppered Steak Slice	170	474.3	13.6	34.3	1.60
Iceland 2 Beef & Vegetable Pasties	360	473.4	13.9	40.3	1.00
Sainsbury's Cheese & Onion Pasty	150	426.0	14.7	33.8	0.80

Suggested Brands	Size (g)	Kcal	S.fat (g)	Carbs (g)	£
Holland's Beef & Veg Pasty	204	554.9	16.3	51.0	1.00
Waitrose premium hand crimped Cornish pasty	200	566.0	16.6	48.0	1.79
Waitrose 1 Cornish Pasty	200	602.0	16.8	52.0	2.00
Waitrose Cheddar hand crimped cheese onion pasty	200	554.0	17.2	52.2	1.79

VALUES SHOWN PER PASTY

Pork Pie

Suggested Brands	Size (g)	Kcal	S.fat (g)	Carbs (g)	£
Tesco Finest 6 Mini Melton Mowbray Pork Pies	300	181.2	4.3	12.2	3.10
Sainsbury's Mini Melton Mowbray Pork Pies	300	203.5	5.7	13.3	1.75
Waitrose 2 Melton Mowbray	150	288.0	7.0	19.5	1.39
ASDA 4 Snack Pork Pies	260	250.9	7.2	17.6	1.50
ASDA Individual Melton Mowbray Pork Pie	140	548.8	12.0	35.0	1.00
Tesco Counter Individual Pork Pie	140	542.5	13.0	37.8	1.50
ASDA 6 Mini Pork Pies	300	203.0	13.5	5.5	1.65
Dickinson & Morris Melton Mowbray Pork Pie	140	537.6	13.7	35.1	1.50
Pork Farms 4 Snack Pork Pies	260	256.1	16.8	21.5	2.00
ASDA Smart Price 4 Large Snack Pork Pies	440	374.0	23.1	31.9	1.20
Morrison's Melton Mowbray Mini Pork Pies	300	1140.0	29.1	82.8	2.00
ASDA Medium Melton Mowbray Pork Pie	295	1126.9	32.5	79.7	2.00
Tesco Large Melton Mowbray Pork Pie	440	1490.7	36.7	97.2	2.50
Waitrose Melton Mowbray large	440	1548.8	42.2	78.8	2.70

SNACKS   PORK PIE

Suggested Brands	Size (g)	Kcal	S.fat (g)	Carbs (g)	£
Sainsbury's Large Melton Mowbray Pork Pie	440	1562.0	42.7	97.2	2.50
Morrison's Large Pork Pie	440	1509.2	43.6	89.3	2.15
Pork Farms Medium Pork Pie	295	1109.2	75.2	79.7	1.85

VALUES SHOWN PER PIE

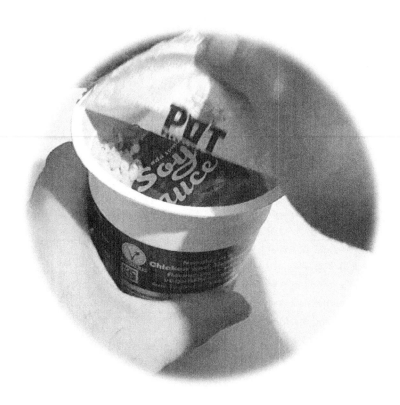

Pot Snacks

Suggested Brands	Size (g)	Kcal	S.fat (g)	Carbs (g)	£
Naked Noodle Soup Ramen Chinese Hot & Sour	80	272	0.1	59.1	1.00
Sainsbury's Rice Noodle Pot Tom Yum	74	273	0.2	59.5	0.50
Batchelors Pasta 'n' Sauce Pot Chicken & Mushroom	65	239	0.3	50.7	1.00
Sharwoods Chicken Chow Mein Noodle Pot	70	253	0.3	46.7	1.50
Naked Noodle Vietnamese Beef Pho	78	267	0,.3	50.1	1.15
Sharwoods Sweet Chilli Chicken Noodle Pot	75	276	0.3	52.0	1.50
ASDA Free From Fiery Chilli Rice Noodle Pot	75	293	0.3	65	1.00
Sharwoods Sweet And Sour Noodle Pot	83	296	0.3	62.3	1.50
ASDA Slimzone Teriyaki Noodle Snack Pot	72	269	0.4	50	0.70
ASDA Free From Chow Mein Rice Noodle Pot	75	290	0.4	63	1.00
ASDA Slimzone Chow Mein Noodle Snack Pot	74	298	0.4	56	0.70
Naked Noodle Singapore Curry	104	359	0.4	70.3	1.00
Sainsbury's Pasta Pot, Tomato & Herb	71	214	0.5	42.2	0.75
ASDA Slimzone Singapore Noodle Snack Pot	71	264	0.5	47	0.70

Suggested Brands	Size (g)	Kcal	S.fat (g)	Carbs (g)	£
ASDA Free From Singapore Curry Rice Noodle Pot	75	283	0.5	61	1.00
Tesco Free From Curry Noodle Pot	74	293	0.5	62.5	1.50
Naked Noodle Egg Noodles Chinese Szechuan	78	294	0.5	57.5	1.15
Naked Noodle Chinese Chow Mein	78	269	0.6	51.7	1.15
Naked Noodle Thai Sweet Chilli	78	271	0.6	52.8	1.15
Naked Noodle Cantonese Hoisin Duck	78	273	0.6	53	1.15
Naked Noodle Malaysian Mee Goreng	104	357	0.6	70.4	1.00
Naked Noodle Japanese Teriyaki	78	265	0.7	51.2	1.15
Naked Noodle Singapore Curry	78	270	0.7	51.8	1.15
Naked Noodle Chinese Firecracker Chicken	78	300	0.7	59.2	1.15
Kabuto Noodles miso ramen pot	85	300	0.9	56	2.00
Kabuto Noodles beef pho pot	85	309	0.9	58	2.00
Kabuto noodles chilli chicken ramen pot	85	327	0.9	60	2.00
John West Steam Pot Tuna Infusions with Jalepenos & Spicy Red Pepper Cous Cous	150	390	1.1	50.4	1.75

Suggested Brands	Size (g)	Kcal	S.fat (g)	Carbs (g)	£
Sainsbury's Pasta Pot, Creamy Chicken	61	233	1.3	42.2	0.75
Naked Noodle Thai Fiery Chicken Panang	104	364	1.3	69.1	1.00
Naked Noodle Egg Noodles Thai Red Curry	78	277	1.6	49.7	1.15
Sainsbury's Rice Pot Chicken Tikka	75	281	1.7	54.2	1.05
Batchelors Pasta 'n' Sauce Pot Mac 'n' Cheese	65	246	1.8	44.7	1.00
Batchelors Pasta 'n' Sauce Pot Cheese & Broccoli	65	247	1.8	45.4	1.00
Batchelors Pasta 'n' Sauce Pot Cheese & Pancetta	65	247	1.8	45.5	1.00
Sainsbury's Rice Noodle Pot Chicken	74	284	1.8	56.4	0.50
Pot Pasta Snack, Tomato Mozzarella	72	258	1.9	46	1.20
Pot Rice Chicken Teriyaki Snack Pot	81	308	2	61	1.00
Pot Rice Chicken Teriyaki Snack	81	308	2.0	61	1.00
Naked Noodle Thai Green Curry	78	305	2.4	53.6	1.15
Naked Noodle Soup Ramen Malaysian Laksa	80	282	3.1	53.2	1.00
Prep Co. Thai Green Curry Rice & Quinoa Pot	68	274	3.3	48	2.00
Naked Noodle Thai Green Curry	104	377	3.5	66	1.00

Suggested Brands	Size (g)	Kcal	S.fat (g)	Carbs (g)	£
Hearty Food Co Spicy Curry Noodle Pot	70	283	3.6	45.3	0.28
Pot Rice Vegetable Curry Snack Pot	87	330	3.7	57	1.00
Pot Rice Vegetable Curry Snack	87	330	3.7	57	1.00
Morrison Chicken & Mushroom Noodle Pot	90	372	3.9	63.3	0.47
Morrison Curry Noodle Pot	90	368	4.0	62.2	0.47
Morrison Beef & Tomato Noodle Pot	90	377	4.1	64.1	0.47
Pot Rice Chicken Risotto Snack Pot	75	288	4.3	48	1.00
Pot Rice Chicken Risotto Snack	75	288	4.3	48	1.00
Prep Co. Indian Spiced Lentils & Rice Po	72	296	4.7	42	2.00
Pot Pasta Macaroni Cheese Snack Pot	62	269	5.8	36	1.00
Pot Pasta Macaroni Cheese Snack	62	269	5.8	36	1.00
Pot Pasta Snack, Cheesy Broccoli	69	288	5.9	38	1.20
Pot Pasta Snack, Creamy Carbonara	62	275	7.1	34	1.20
Batchelors Super Noodles Chicken	75	353	7.5	47	1.00
Batchelors Super Noodles Flamin' Curry	77	360	7.5	47.7	1.00

Suggested Brands	Size (g)	Kcal	S.fat (g)	Carbs (g)	£
Batchelors Super Noodles Sweet & Sour	82	379	7.5	53.5	1.00
Batchelors Super Noodles Curry	75	351	7.6	46.1	1.00
Batchelors Super Noodles Bacon	75	351	7.6	46.4	1.00
Batchelors Super Noodles BBQ Beef	75	354	7.6	46.5	1.00
Batchelors Super Noodles Sweet Chilli	79	368	7.6	50.6	1.00
Pot Noodle Pulled Pork	90	426	7.6	61	1.00
Pot Noodle Chinese Chow Mein	90	430	7.9	58	1.00
Pot Noodle Sticky Rib	90	461	8.2	65	1.00
Pot Noodle Original Curry	90	471	8.4	67	1.00
Pot Noodle Beef & Tomato	90	461	8.5	62	1.00
Pot Noodle Bombay Bad Boy	90	463	8.5	63	1.00
Pot Noodle Sweet & Sour	90	466	8.5	66	1.00
Pot Noodle Chilli Beef	90	461	8.6	62	1.00
Pot Noodle Chicken Korma	90	463	8.6	62	1.00
Pot Noodle Chicken & Mushroom	90	459	9.0	62.7	1.00

Values Shown Per Prepared Pot

Sausage Rolls

Suggested Brands	Size (g)	Kcal	S.fat (g)	Carbs (g)	£
Tesco 20 Mini Sausage	220	34.0	0.8	3.2	2.00
Sainsbury's Sausage Mini Rolls x20	310	50.5	1.3	4.3	2.15
Wall's 12 Cocktail Pork	240	68.0	2.0	4.1	1.00
Morrisons 9 Three Bird Sausage	288	94.1	2.2	6.7	2.00
ASDA 12 Snack Cheese & Onion	360	88.8	2.3	9.0	1.25
Tesco 9 Snack Sausage	270	94.5	2.5	7.6	1.75
ASDA 9 Pork & Chorizo	279	108.8	2.9	8.1	1.50
ASDA 12 Snack Pork	372	111.6	3.4	8.1	1.25
6 Pork Sausage	360	154.8	3.4	14.8	1.59
Quorn 3 Sausage Rolls	210	181.3	3.7	17.2	2.25
ASDA 30% Reduced Fat Pork x6	360	172.8	3.9	16.8	1.50
Sainsbury's Sausage Rolls, Basics x6	300	164.5	4.0	14.6	1.15
Linda McCartney Sausage	342	163.6	4.2	12.9	1.93
ASDA Smart Price 8 Pork	480	195.6	4.8	19.2	0.99
Wall's 4 Pork	240	187.2	4.9	15.7	1.75
Sainsbury's Cheese & Onion Rolls x6	396	150.5	5.0	20.2	1.80
Tesco 6 Sausage	360	189.0	5.0	15.2	1.75
Sainsbury's Sausage Rolls x6	360	199.2	5.0	16.9	1.80
ASDA 6 Pork	360	226.2	6.6	17.4	1.25
ASDA Cumberland Sausage	360	226.2	6.6	16.2	1.50

Snacks Sausage Rolls

Suggested Brands	Size (g)	Kcal	S.fat (g)	Carbs (g)	£
Morrisons The Best Pork & Caramelised Onion	188	208.7	7.0	13.0	2.20
Genius Gluten Free Sausage x2	200	261.0	8.2	21.8	2.20
Birds Eye 4 Home Baked	360	284.4	8.2	21.6	1.50
Shazans Select 2 Sausage	260	367.9	11.6	33.6	2.00
Greggs 4 Sausage	427	338.4	12.8	24.6	1.69

Values Shown Per Sausage Roll

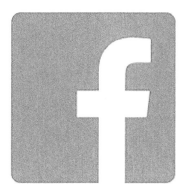

www.facebook.com/StephenDBarnes

Scotch Eggs

Suggested Brands	Size (g)	Kcal	S.fat (g)	Carbs (g)	£
Quorn mini savoury eggs (12)	240	50.0	0.3	3.6	2.00
ASDA Savoury Egg Bites (8)	84	29.8	0.4	2.6	0.75
ASDA Sharing 18 Savoury Egg Bites	216	34.1	0.5	3.0	1.65
ASDA Sharing 18 Savoury Egg Bites	216	34.1	0.5	3.0	1.65
Sainsbury's Egg Bites, Mini x6	72	34.2	0.6	2.5	0.75
Sainsbury's Egg Bites, Mini x18	216	34.2	0.6	2.5	2.00
Morrisons Mini Scotch Eggs (18)	216	43.7	0.6	3.3	1.95
ASDA 12 Mini Savoury Eggs	216	51.1	0.7	4.5	1.00
Tesco Mini Savoury Eggs 12 Pack	216	50.9	0.8	3.5	1.00
Quorn Meat Free Picnic Eggs (3)	180	150.0	0.8	10.9	1.50
Iceland 12 Mini Savoury Eggs	216	49.5	0.9	3.3	1.00
Morrisons Mini Savoury Scotch Eggs 12 Pack	216	59.4	0.9	4.5	1.00
Sainsbury's Egg Bites x6	120	56.4	1.0	3.9	0.70
Sainsbury's Egg Bites x12	240	56.4	1.0	3.9	1.00
essential Waitrose 12 picnic eggs	240	56.4	1.0	3.8	1.35

Suggested Brands	Size (g)	Kcal	S.fat (g)	Carbs (g)	£
Quorn Mini Savoury Eggs (3)	240	200.0	1.1	14.6	2.00
Sainsbury's Mini Savoury Eggs, Taste the Difference x8	200	83.8	1.7	2.8	2.50
Waitrose 1 Soft Poached Scotch Egg	120	256.8	3.7	9.0	2.09
ASDA 2 Cumberland Scotch Eggs	226	241.8	3.8	17.0	1.00
Wall's Classic Scotch Eggs x2	226	310.8	4.0	14.5	1.10
Free Range Scotch Egg with Sausagemeat (1)	140	299.6	4.3	10.5	1.19
ASDA Extra Special Runny Scotch Eggs (2)	226	254.3	4.5	10.2	2.50
ASDA 4 Scotch Eggs	452	266.7	4.6	18.1	1.65
ASDA 2 Ploughmans Scotch Eggs	226	273.5	4.6	18.1	1.00
Tesco Scotch Eggs 4 Pack	454	266.7	4.9	16.9	1.65
Sainsbury's Scotch Eggs x4	452	45.2	5.2	16.7	1.95
Sainsbury's Individual Scotch Egg (1)	113	271.2	5.2	16.7	0.60
Sainsbury's Scotch Eggs x2	226	271.2	5.2	16.7	1.00
Tesco Deli Scotch Egg (1)	120	282.0	5.2	17.9	0.50
Tesco Finest 2 Scotch Eggs	240	301.2	5.2	11.9	2.00
Iceland 2 Scotch Eggs	226	287.0	5.3	18.8	1.00
Morrisons Scotch Eggs 4 Pack	452	306.2	5.5	20.0	1.70
Free Range Scotch Egg with Chorizo & Red Pepper (1)	140	333.2	6.2	11.8	1.19

SNACKS   SCOTCH EGGS

Suggested Brands	Size (g)	Kcal	S.fat (g)	Carbs (g)	£
essential Waitrose 2 scotch eggs	246	334.6	7.0	16.7	1.09
Waitrose Succulent scotch egg (1)	140	438.2	10.2	11.2	1.39
Seasonal Scotch Egg Chorizo & Parsley (1)	140	540.4	10.2	25.3	1.41
Sainsbury's Scotch Egg, Taste the Difference (1)	180	543.6	12.2	14.8	1.30

VALUES SHOWN PER EGG

Your Favourite Food Not Included?
Let Us Know

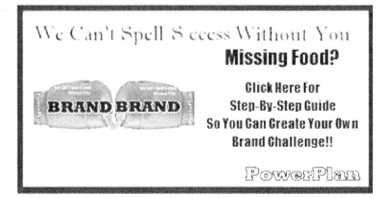

WWW.WECANTSPELLSUCCESSWITHOUTYOU.COM

Steak and Kidney Pie

Suggested Brands	Size (g)	Kcal	S.fat (g)	Carbs (g)	£
Fray Bentos Classic Steak & Kidney Pie	425	544.0	6.0	63.8	1.00
Holland's 4 Steak & Kidney Pies	600	403.0	7.4	40.0	2.00
ASDA 4 Steak & Kidney Pies	600	352.5	7.7	31.5	2.07
Morrisons 4 Steak & Kidney Pies	600	340.5	7.8	31.5	2.00
Sainsbury's Steak & Kidney Puff Pastry Pie	150	378.0	8.4	33.6	0.75
Pukka Pies Steak & Kidney Pie	238	537.0	11.2	42.3	1.65
Pieminister Kate & Sidney Pie	270	545.4	11.6	58.9	3.70
Princes Steak & Kidney Pie	425	569.5	12.8	55.3	1.00
Tesco Steak And Kidney Shortcrust Pie	200	546.0	13.4	47.2	1.50
ASDA Slow Cooked Steak & Kidney Puff Pastry Pie	200	556.0	13.8	44.0	1.28

VALUES SHOWN PER PIE

Notes

Drinks

Try to select a low or no sugar diet drink. A typical cola drink will contain 105 calories per 250 ml glass and 27 grams of sugar. A diet cola drink will only contain 2 calories per 250 ml glass and less than 0.5 grams of sugar. The diet option will help with weight control along with the avoidance of excessive sugar that could lead to diabetes type 2.

When suffering from stomach issues, such as IBS, it is better to drink tea, coffee and fruit juice. Using fizzy drinks will only irritate the condition over time.

When drinking tea or coffee do not count calories, when using sweeteners rather than sugar, as there are only a few calories in the drink.

Always include calories from hot chocolate, latte, cappuccino, milkshake, smoothies and general drinks from either the supermarket or coffee vendors.

Coffee

(Cappuccino, Latte, Instant And Filter)

Suggested Brands	Size (g)	Kcal	S.fat (g)	Carbs (g)	£
Standard Instant Coffee	200	2.4	0.0	0.1	2.10
Nescafe Azera Americano Instant Coffe	100	2.4	0.0	0.0	2.74
Nescafe Azera Intenso Instant Coffee	100	2.4	0.0	0.0	2.74
Nescafe Gold Blend Instant Coffee	200	2.4	0.0	0.1	4.00
Nescafe Gold Smooth Instant Coffee	200	2.4	0.0	0.1	4.00
Nescafe Original Instant Coffee	300	2.4	0.0	0.1	4.50
ASDA Skinny Latte Coffee Pods. Dolce Gusto Compatible	16 pack	49.4	0.0	7.8	2.89
Alpro Caffè Coffee & Soya Caramel Drink	235	82.3	0.2	11.5	1.00
ASDA Café Au Lait Coffee Pods. Dolce Gusto Compatible	16 pack	49.4	0.7	6.3	2.89
ASDA Flat White Coffee Pods. Dolce Gusto Compatible	16 pack	58.8	0.7	8.7	2.89
Sainsbury's Instant Skinny Latte	144	70.5	0.9	9.9	1.00
Morrisons Instant Mocha Coffee Sachets	128	70.5	1.2	12.9	1.30
Nescafe Latte Cafe Menu Latte Skiny	156	70.5	1.2	10.6	1.50

Suggested Brands	Size (g)	Kcal	S.fat (g)	Carbs (g)	£
Morrisons Instant Cappuccino Unsweetened Sachets	128	70.5	1.4	12.7	1.30
Nescafe Cafe Menu Vanilla	148	72.9	1.4	12.9	1.50
Starbucks Skinny Latte	220	82.3	1.4	9.4	1.00
Nescafe Gold Cappuccino Unsweetened	113.6	51.7	1.6	7.1	1.50
Sainsbury's Instant Cappuccino	136	79.9	1.6	13.2	1.00
Sainsbury's Instant Mocha	160	89.3	1.6	15.7	1.00
Nescafe Gold Cappuccino Decaffeinated Unsweetened	120	58.8	1.9	7.8	1.50
Morrisons Instant Cappuccino Sweetened Coffee Sachets	128	75.2	1.9	12.9	1.30
Sainsbury's Instant Latte	144	82.3	1.9	12.5	1.00
Nescafe Original 3 In 1	136	84.6	1.9	15.3	1.89
Tassimo 8 Kenco Mocha Coffee Pods	8x26	124.6	1.9	21.2	3.99
Tassimo 8 Costa Cappuccino Pods	280	49.4	2.0	2.8	4.00
Tassimo Costa Cappuccino Coffee	8 pods	49.4	2.0	2.8	4.00
Tassimo 8 Costa Caramel Latte Pods	271	61.1	2.0	7.8	4.00
Tassimo 8 L'OR Latte Macchiato Skinny Coffee Pods	264	40.0	2.1	3.5	4.49
Tassimo 8 Kenco Cappuccino Pods	260	58.8	2.1	5.2	3.99

DRINKS COFFEE

Suggested Brands	Size (g)	Kcal	S.fat (g)	Carbs (g)	£
Tassimo 8 Costa Vanilla Latte Pods	271	65.8	2.1	8.5	4.00
ASDA Cappuccino Coffee 8 Milk Pods & 8 Coffee Pods. Dolce Gusto Compatible	16 pack	79.9	2.1	8.5	2.89
Starbucks Discoveries Qandi Caramel	220	141.0	2.1	21.2	1.00
Tassimo 8 Costa Latte Pods	239	47.0	2.3	3.8	4.00
Tassimo Costa Latte Coffee Pods	8 pods	51.7	2.4	4.2	4.00
Tassimo 8 Espresso Caramel Latte Macchiato Pods	271	65.8	2.4	8.5	4.49
Tassimo 8 Baileys Latte Macchiato Coffee Pods	264	75.2	2.6	8.9	4.00
ASDA Latte Coffee 8 Milk Pods & 8 Coffee Pods Dolce Gusto Compatible	16 pack	94.0	2.8	8.7	2.89
Tassimo 8 L'OR Espresso Latte Macchiato Pods	267	75.2	3.8	5.9	4.49
Starbucks Fairtrade DoubleShot Espresso No Added Sugar	200	117.5	3.8	9.2	1.00
Starbucks Caffe-Latte	220	164.5	4.0	20.9	1.00

VALUES SHOWN PER 235ML CUP

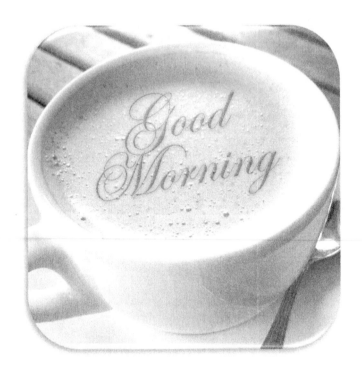

Cola

Suggested Brands	Size (g)	Kcal	S.fat (g)	Carbs (g)	£
Coca-Cola Zero Sugar	1.25	0.9	0.0	0.0	1.00
Coca-Cola Zero Sugar Vanilla	1.25	0.9	0.0	0.0	1.00
Diet Coke Exotic Mango	1.25	0.9	0.0	0.0	1.00
essential Waitrose sugar-free diet cola	2	0.9	0.0	0.3	1.05
Diet Coke	1.25	1.1	0.0	0.0	1.00
Coca-Cola Zero Sugar Peach	1.25	1.1	0.0	0.0	1.00
Coca-Cola Zero Sugar Raspberry	1.25	1.1	0.0	0.0	1.00
Tesco Craft Cola Botanical	1	1.4	0.0	0.0	0.45
Tesco Craft Cola Coffee	1	1.4	0.0	0.3	0.45
Tesco Diet Cola	2	1.4	0.0	0.3	0.50
Tesco Xero Cola Cherry	2	1.4	0.0	0.3	0.50
Tesco Classic Diet Caffeine Free Cola	2	1.4	0.0	0.3	0.89
Diet Coke Twisted Strawberry	1.25	1.4	0.0	0.0	1.00
Pepsi Max Raspberry	1.25	1.4	0.0	0.3	1.00
Pepsi Max Cherry	1.25	1.7	0.0	0.0	1.00
Pepsi Max Ginger	1.25	1.7	0.0	0.3	1.00
Sainsbury's Cola Zero	2	2.8	0.0	0.6	0.45
Sainsbury's Diet Cola	2	2.8	0.0	0.6	0.45
ASDA Diet Cola	2	2.8	0.0	0.3	0.50
ASDA Diet Cola Caffeine Free	2	2.8	0.0	0.6	0.50
Morrisons No Added Sugar Diet Cola	2	2.8	0.0	0.6	0.60

DRINKS   COLA

Suggested Brands	Size (g)	Kcal	S.fat (g)	Carbs (g)	£
Pepsi Max	2	11.4	0.0	0.0	1.20
Barr Cola	2	39.8	0.0	10.2	1.00
Sainsbury's Cola	2	56.8	0.0	14.2	0.45
ASDA Cola	2	56.8	0.0	13.9	0.50
Morrisons Cola	2	56.8	0.0	14.2	0.60
Fentimans Curiosity Cola	0.25	96.6	0.0	22.2	1.10
essential Waitrose cola	2	113.6	0.0	28.4	1.49
Pepsi Regular	2	116.4	0.0	31.2	2.00
Coca-Cola Classic Bottle	1.25	119.3	0.0	0.0	1.79
Coca Cola Classic	1.5	119.3	0.0	30.1	1.95
Coca-Cola Classic Cherry	1.5	127.8	0.0	31.8	1.95
Tesco Xero Cola	2	1.4	0.1	0.3	0.50
Tesco Cola	2	54.0	0.1	13.6	0.50

VALUES SHOWN PER 284 ML GLASS

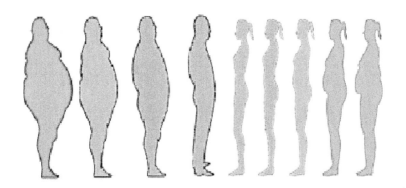

Energy Drinks

Suggested Brands	Size (g)	Kcal	S.fat (g)	Carbs (g)	£
Tiger Energy	250	105.0	0.0	24.5	0.50
Oshee Vitamin Energy Mint-Lime-Lemon Flavour **	250	225.0	0.0	55.0	0.50
Black Energy Drink Mojito	250	100.0	0.0	23.5	0.60
Oshee Vitamin & Mineral Energy Drink **	250	225.0	0.0	55.0	0.60
Black Energy Drink Classic	250	100.0	0.0	24.0	0.65
Sunsoul Energy Drink Natural Passion Fruit	250	160.0	0.0	37.5	0.70
ASDA Diet Blue Charge Stimulation	1000	25.0	0.0	1.0	0.79
Tesco Blue Spark Original	1000	105.0	0.0	24.0	0.79
ASDA Original Blue Charge Stimulation	1000	120.0	0.0	25.0	0.79
Carabao Green Apple Energy	330	95.0	0.0	22.5	0.90
Carabao Mandarin Orange Energy	330	95.0	0.0	22.5	0.90
V Energy Drink	250	105.0	0.0	23.5	0.99
Warrior Power Unleashed Energy Drink x 4	250	80.0	0.0	17.5	1.00
Morrisons Original Source 1899	1000	115.0	0.0	25.0	1.00
Lucozade Energy Wild Cherry	1000	170.0	0.0	42.0	1.00
Lucozade Energy Apple Blast	1000	175.0	0.0	42.0	1.00
Lucozade Energy Orange	1000	175.0	0.0	42.0	1.00

Suggested Brands	Size (g)	Kcal	S.fat (g)	Carbs (g)	£
Lucozade Energy The Brazilian Mango	1000	175.0	0.0	42.5	1.00
Lucozade Energy Caribbean Crush	1000	180.0	0.0	43.5	1.00
Lucozade Energy Original	1000	185.0	0.0	44.5	1.00
Red Bull	250	230.0	0.0	55.0	1.00
Oshee Lime-Mint Flavour Isotonic	750	115.0	0.0	27.0	1.20
Oshee Orange Flavour Isotonic	750	120.0	0.0	27.0	1.20
Oshee Multifruit Flavour Isotonic	750	120.0	0.0	28.5	1.20
Coke Energy	250	210.0	0.0	51.5	1.25
Red Bull Tropical Edition Energy	250	230.0	0.0	55.0	1.25
Tesco Isotonic Sports Drink Raspberry x 4	500	115.0	0.0	26.5	1.26
Tenzing Energy Drink Raspberry & Yuzu	250	95.0	0.0	22.5	1.29
Scheckter's energy lite *	250	100.0	0.0	20.0	1.35
Purdey's Rejuvenate Natural Energy	330	150.0	0.0	31.5	1.35
Scheckter's organic energy *	250	155.0	0.0	35.0	1.35
Scheckter's Ginger Energy *	250	165.0	0.0	40.0	1.45
Tesco Blue Spark Energy x 6	250	120.0	0.0	25.5	1.50
Mountain Dew Energy Drink **	1000	240.0	0.0	65.0	1.80
ASDA Diet Blue Charge x 8	250	25.0	0.0	2.0	2.00

DRINKS ENERGY DRINKS

Suggested Brands	Size (g)	Kcal	S.fat (g)	Carbs (g)	£
Morrisons Original Source 1899 x 6	250	115.0	0.0	25.0	2.00
Kx No Added Sugar Carnival Energy x 4	500	25.0	0.0	3.5	2.50
Kx No Added Sugar Live Energy	500	25.0	0.0	3.5	2.50
Tesco Kx Energy x 4	500	90.0	0.0	20.5	2.50
Lucozade Energy Cherry x 6	380	170.0	0.0	42.0	2.50
Rockstar Punched Guava Energy x 4	500	110.0	0.0	24.5	3.50
Lucozade Sport Raspberry x 6	500	135.0	0.0	32.0	3.50
Lucozade Sport Orange x 6	500	140.0	0.0	32.5	3.50
Lucozade Energy Orange x 8	380	175.0	0.0	42.0	3.50
Lucozade Energy Original x 8	380	185.0	0.0	44.5	3.50
Monster Energy x 4	500	235.0	0.0	60.0	4.00
Red Bull x 8	250	230.0	0.0	55.0	7.50
Monster Energy x 8	500	235.0	0.0	60.0	7.75
Tesco Blue Spark Sugar Free Energy	1000	5.0	0.0	0.0	0.79
Coke Energy No Sugar	250	5.0	0.0	0.0	1.00
Tesco Blue Spark Sugar Free Energy x 6	250	5.0	0.0	0.0	1.50
Monster Energy Ultra Sugar Free	500	10.0	0.0	4.5	1.25
Kx Sugar Free Energy x 4	500	10.0	0.0	0.0	2.50
Kx Sugar Free Ice Energy x 4	500	10.0	0.0	0.0	2.50

Suggested Brands	Size (g)	Kcal	S.fat (g)	Carbs (g)	£
Monster Energy Ultra x 8	500	10.0	0.0	4.5	6.75
Monster Energy Ultra Violet x 4	500	13.0	0.0	7.0	3.50
ASDA Blue Charge Diet Summer Fruits Stimulation	250	15.0	0.0	1.0	0.45
Morrisons Original Source 1899 Sugar Free	1000	15.0	0.0	0.5	1.00
Muscle Moose - Moose Juice Extreme Energy	500	15.0	0.0	1.7	1.75
Muscle Moose - Moose Juice Extreme Energy - Berry Flavour	500	15.0	0.0	1.7	1.75
Muscle Moose - Moose Juice Extreme Energy - Green Apple	500	15.0	0.0	1.7	1.75
Red Bull Sugar Free x 8	250	15.0	0.0	0.0	7.00
ASDA Sport Orange Flavour Isotonic x 4	500	135.0	0.3	32.0	1.26

Values Shown Per 500 ml serving

* Shown As KJ Not Calories On Waitrose Website

** Subject To Sugar Tax

Fruit Tea

Suggested Brands	Size (g)	Kcal	S.fat (g)	Carbs (g)	£
Tetley Super Green Tea Boost Strawberry & Raspberry	20	3	0.0	1.0	1.50
Pukka Elderberry & Echinacea	20	3	0.0	1.0	2.00
Tetley Green Tea with Lemon	50	3	0.0	1.0	2.15
ASDA Strawberry & Forest Fruits	20	7	0.0	2.0	0.74
Twinings Lemon & Ginger	20	7	0.0	0.0	1.50
Twinings Cranberry & Raspberry	20	7	0.0	0.0	1.50
Twinings Spiced Ginger	20	7	0.0	0.0	1.50
Tetley Super Fruits Boost Blueberry & Raspberry Tea Bags	20	7	0.0	2.0	1.50
Twinings Strawberry & Raspberry	20	7	0.0	0.0	1.70
Sainsbury's Cold Brew Watermelon & Lime Flavour	15	7	0.0	0.0	2.50
Sainsbury's Mint Lemonade Cold Brew	15	7	0.0	0.0	2.50
Sainsbury's Cold Brew Peach & Black Tea	15	7	0.0	0.0	2.50
Teapigs super fruit	15	7	0.0	2.0	3.00
ASDA Lemon Meringue	20	1	0.2	0.2	0.74
Twinings Superblends Sleep Spiced Apple &	20	3	0.2	0.2	2.00

Drinks   Fruit Tea

Suggested Brands	Size (g)	Kcal	S.fat (g)	Carbs (g)	£
Vanilla with Camomile & Passionflowers					
Twinings Superblends Glow Strawberry & Cucumber	20	3	0.2	0.2	2.00
ASDA Rhubarb & Custard	20	7	0.2	0.2	0.74
Tesco Red Berries	20	13	0.3	0.3	0.75

Values Shown Per 235ml Cup

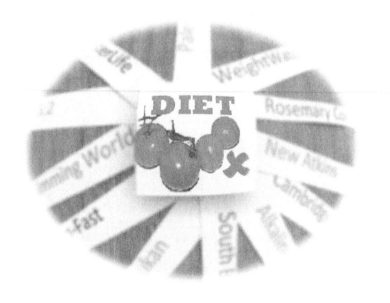

Hot Chocolate

(Instant)

Suggested Brands	Size (g)	Kcal	S.fat (g)	Carbs (g)	£
Galaxy Drinking Chocolate	500	66.8	0.3	13.9	2.50
Sweet Freedom Choc Shot	320	48.2	0.4	9.4	3.00
Twinings Swiss	350	70.0	0.4	14.6	3.00
Sainsbury's Basics Fairtrade	400	68.2	0.5	14.0	1.00
ASDA Smart Price Instant	400	70.0	0.5	15.0	0.79
Cadbury 30% Less Sugar	280	60.7	0.6	7.9	2.00
ASDA Instant	400	72.0	0.6	14.1	1.04
Cadbury Wispa Frothy Instant	246	71.5	0.7	13.3	2.00
Cadbury Drinking	250	72.4	0.7	13.7	1.99
Options Mint Madness	220	63.0	0.8	9.5	4.00
ASDA Reduced Sugar Instant	300	68.6	0.8	11.1	1.39
Green & Black's Organic	300	70.9	0.8	12.1	3.59
Cadbury Freddo	290	72.4	0.8	13.7	2.50
Options Belgian Chocolate	220	66.1	0.9	9.5	4.00
Ovaltine Light	300	67.7	0.9	13.3	3.00
Maltesers Malty	350	70.7	0.9	14.0	2.59
Clipper Fairtrade	250	71.1	0.9	11.7	2.50
Options Hot Chocolate Salted Caramel	220	62.5	1.0	9.2	4.00
San Cristobal Rich	250	68.4	1.0	11.6	3.00
Sainsbury's Instant Fairtrade	350	68.6	1.0	12.2	1.70
Sainsbury's Low Calorie Instant Fairtrade	250	65.5	1.2	9.3	1.50
Galaxy Frothy Top Instant	275	69.7	1.2	13.0	2.58

DRINKS   HOT CHOCOLATE

Suggested Brands	Size (g)	Kcal	S.fat (g)	Carbs (g)	£
Cadbury Oreo	260	73.1	1.2	12.8	2.00
Aero Instant	288	73.3	1.2	13.4	2.99
Options White Chocolate	220	72.4	1.4	12.8	4.00
Cadbury Highlights Milk	220	62.5	1.7	6.7	3.99
Galaxy Light Style Instant	180	68.9	1.8	9.5	2.00
Lucy Bee Organic	250	69.5	1.9	2.8	4.00
Tesco Finest Santo Domingo	250	154.8	3.2	17.9	2.50

VALUES SHOWN PER 18 GRAMS OF POWDER WITH HOT WATER

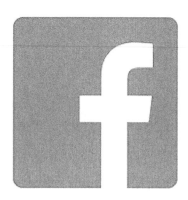

www.facebook.com/StephendDBarnes

Lemonade

Suggested Brands	Size (g)	Kcal	S.fat (g)	Carbs (g)	£
ASDA Smart Price Lemonade	2000	1.3	0.0	0.0	0.17
Morrisons Diet Lemonade	2000	2.5	0.0	0.0	0.60
Sprite Zero	2000	2.5	0.0	0.0	1.85
Geebee Free the Fizz Lemonade No Added Sugar	2000	2.5	0.0	0.0	0.50
Tesco No Added Sugar Cloudy Lemonade	2000	5.0	0.0	0.1	0.50
Schweppes Slimline Lemonade	2000	5.0	0.0	0.0	1.00
R Whites Diet Lemonade	2000	5.0	0.0	0.0	1.30
7UP Free Sparkling Lemon & Lime	2000	5.0	0.0	0.0	1.50
Lucozade Zero Pink Lemonade	1000	6.3	0.0	0.3	1.00
Waitrose lemonade with lemon juice no added sugar	1000	7.5	0.0	0.5	0.66
Tesco Sparkling Morello Cherry Lemonade	1000	7.5	0.0	1.0	0.45
C&C Lemonade	2000	22.5	0.0	4.8	1.50
R Whites Lemonade	1500	27.5	0.0	6.0	0.70
Barr Lemonade	2000	30.0	0.0	7.0	0.75
Morrisons Lemonade	2000	32.5	0.0	7.5	0.60
Sprite Original	2000	35.0	0.0	8.3	1.85
Fever-Tree Refreshingly Light Sicilian Lemonade	500	42.5	0.0	10.5	1.70

Suggested Brands	Size (g)	Kcal	S.fat (g)	Carbs (g)	£
R Whites Premium Pear & Elderflower Lemonade	1250	42.5	0.0	9.8	1.00
R Whites Premium Raspberry Lemonade	1250	42.5	0.0	9.8	1.00
Schweppes Lemonade	2000	45.0	0.0	10.5	1.00
Waitrose Duchy Rose Lemonade	750	45.0	0.0	11.5	2.29
Fanta Lemon	2000	47.5	0.0	11.3	1.85
Belvoir Fruit Farms Fruit Farms Raspberry Lemonade	750	75.0	0.0	18.8	2.49
Belvoir Fruit Farms Fruit Farms Raspberry Lemonade	750	75.0	0.0	18.8	2.49
Fairtrade Lemony Lemonade	330	101.5	0.0	24.4	1.69
Fentimans Traditional Rose Lemonade	750	102.5	0.0	23.0	2.95
Nash Red Lemonade	1500	220.0	0.0	12.3	1.37
Sainsbury's Diet Lemonade	2000	2.5	0.1	0.0	0.70
essential Waitrose sugar free lemonade	2000	2.5	0.1	0.0	0.72
ASDA Diet Lemonade	2000	2.5	0.1	0.0	0.35
Tesco Sparkling Diet Lemonade	2000	2.5	0.1	0.0	0.35
Waitrose cloudy lemonade light	2000	5.0	0.1	0.5	0.81
Tesco Sparkling Raspberry And Rose Lemonade	1000	5.0	0.1	0.1	0.45

Suggested Brands	Size (g)	Kcal	S.fat (g)	Carbs (g)	£
Tesco Sparkling Watermelon Lemonade	1000	5.0	0.1	0.5	0.45
ASDA Diet Cloudy Lemonade	2000	5.0	0.1	0.3	0.50
Sainsbury's Cloudy Lemonade No Added Sugar	2000	7.5	0.1	0.5	0.70
Tesco No Added Sugar Pink Lemonade	2000	7.5	0.1	0.8	0.50
Sainsbury's Pink Lemonade, Zero Added Sugar	2000	10.0	0.1	0.3	1.00
Morrisons The Best Sparkling Raspberry Lemonade	750	10.0	0.1	2.3	1.50
ASDA Lemonade	2000	25.0	0.1	5.8	0.35
Tesco Sparkling Lemonade	2000	30.0	0.1	7.3	0.35
Sainsbury's Lemonade	2000	37.5	0.1	8.8	0.70
ASDA Extra Special Freshly Squeezed Cloudy Lemonade	1000	60.0	0.1	0.8	2.00
Waitrose lemonade with lemon juice	1000	75.0	0.1	17.5	0.89
Waitrose cloudy lemonade	2000	80.0	0.1	19.5	1.24
Waitrose 1 freshly squeezed still lemonade	1000	85.0	0.1	19.5	2.65
Sainsbury's Sicilian Lemonade, Sparkling, Taste the Difference(Sugar levy applied)	750	85.0	0.1	20.3	2.00

Suggested Brands	Size (g)	Kcal	S.fat (g)	Carbs (g)	£
Morrisons The Best Sparkling Sicilian Lemonade	750	120.0	0.1	27.8	1.50

VALUES SHOWN PER 250ML GLASS

Malt Drinks

Suggested Brands	Size (g)	Kcal	S.fat (g)	Carbs (g)	£
Horlicks Instant Light	500	117	0.5	22.5	3.50
ASDA Instant	400	131	0.9	26	1.49
Horlicks Instant Light Chocolate	500	117	1.4	22	3.50
Sainsbury's Instant	400	130	2	23.1	1.30
Horlicks Traditional Malt	500	241	3.5	36	3.50
Tesco Malted	300	259	3.8	40.2	1.15

VALUES SHOWN PER 32 GRAMS OF POWDER WITH HOT WATER

Tea (Black)

Suggested Brands	Size (g)	Kcal	S.fat (g)	Carbs (g)	£
PG Tips	240	1.2	0.0	0.0	3.50
Scottish Blend Original	200	1.2	0.0	0.0	3.79
PG Tips Decaf	180	1.2	0.0	0.0	4.00
Sainsbury's Fairtrade SO Organic	80	2.4	0.0	0.5	1.50
Sainsbury's Fairly Traded Gold Label	80	2.4	0.0	0.2	1.75
Tetley	80	2.4	0.0	0.7	2.65
Tetley Extra Strong	75	2.4	0.0	0.7	2.85
Clipper Everyday Organic	100	2.4	0.0	0.5	3.00
Tetley Decaf	160	2.4	0.0	0.7	3.00
Clipper Everyday Fair Trade	100	2.4	0.0	0.0	3.50
Yorkshire Tea *	160	2.4	0.0	0.0	5.39
Typhoo	900	2.4	0.0	0.0	9.00
Sainsbury's basics	100	2.4	0.2	0.5	0.50
ssential Waitrose Original Blend Decaffeinated	80	2.4	0.2	0.5	1.59
Essential Waitrose Original Blend	160	2.4	0.2	0.5	2.10
Asda everyday *	80	7.3	0.2	0.5	0.89
Asda everyday decaf *	80	7.3	0.2	0.5	0.89
Twinings English Breakfast *`	50	7.3	0.2	0.5	2.00
Yorkshire Tea Decaf *	160	7.3	0.2	0.5	5.00
Stockwell & Co *	80	7.4	0.2	0.5	0.58
Tesco Tea	80	7.4	0.2	0.5	0.89
Morrisons Everyday *	80	7.4	0.2	0.5	1.25
Asda Extra Strong *	80	7.4	0.2	0.5	1.39

Suggested Brands	Size (g)	Kcal	S.fat (g)	Carbs (g)	£
Lancashire Tea Foil Fresh *	80	7.4	0.2	0.5	1.50
Tesco Decaffeinated	80	7.4	0.2	0.5	1.50
Tesco Gold	80	7.4	0.2	0.5	1.69
Thompson's Special Everyday *	160	7.4	0.2	0.5	3.00
Morrisons Extra Strong *	80	7.5	0.2	0.5	1.65
Morrisons Decaffeinated *	160	7.5	0.2	0.5	3.15

VALUES SHOWN PER 235ML CUP

* NUTRITION NOT SHOWN ON WEBSITE

Tonic Water

Suggested Brands	Size (g)	Kcal	S.fat (g)	Carbs (g)	£
ASDA Diet Indian With Lime	1000	12	0	0	0.37
Tesco Low Calorie Indian	1000	15	0	0	0.40
ASDA Diet Indian	1000	16	0	0	0.37
Morrison's Diet Indian	1000	16	0	0	0.45
Sainsbury's Diet Indian	1000	16	0	0	0.50
Waitrose sugar free indian	1000	16	0	0	0.53
Tesco Diet Indian With Lime	1000	19.2	0	0.28	0.40
ASDA Diet Indian With Lemon	1000	20	0	0	0.37
Schweppes Slimline	1000	20	0	0	1.22
Tesco Diet Indian With Lemon	1000	22.8	0	0.28	0.40

Drinks

Suggested Brands	Size (g)	Kcal	S.fat (g)	Carbs (g)	£
Morrison's Diet Indian With Lime	1000	24	0	0	0.45
Morrison's Diet Indian With Lemon	1000	24	0	0	0.45
Fever-Tree Naturally Light	500	75	0	19	1.70
Fever-Tree Premium	500	140	0	35.5	1.81
Morrison's Indian	1000	152	0	34.4	0.45
Tesco Indian	1000	158.4	0	36	0.40
Fever-Tree Elderflower	500	170	0	42.5	1.81
Fever Tree Mediterranean	500	180	0	45	1.81
Sainsbury's Indian	1000	204	0	48	0.50
Waitrose indian	1000	208	0	49.2	0.53
Schweppes Tonic water	1000	212	0	48	1.22
Llanllyr Source (4 x 200ml)	800	264	0	64	3.99
ASDA Indian	1000	136	0.3	29.6	0.37

Values Shown Per 284 ml Glass

Notes

Alcohol

You will need to count all the calories from alcoholic drinks, along with food, and add them to the number of calories consumed during the day.

Try a low sugar alcoholic drink when relaxing at night to avoid excessive sugar being converted to fat when consumed late at night. Selecting a drink high in sugar, like red wine, is a sure way of increasing your weight that could also result in a diabetes type 2 diagnosis over time.

Be aware when reducing your daily calorie count, any alcoholic drinks will have a greater impact on the body. This will result in you feeling intoxicated very quickly that will impair your judgement.

Ale

Suggested Brands	Size (ml)	Kcal	S.fat (g)	Carbs (g)	£
Brewdog Nanny State Alcohol Free Hoppy Ale x 4	300	78.0	0.0	3.0	4.00
Shipyard Low Tide Pale Ale	500	85.0	0.0	15.9	1.30
Hyde & Wilde Pale Ale	330	141.9	0.0	10.2	1.50
Sainsbury's Rye Pale Ale	500	145.0	0.0	15.5	1.50
Tetley's Smooth Ale	440	145.2	0.0	11.9	0.67
Bass British Pale Ale	355	163.3	0.0	11.0	1.70
Whitstable Bay Pale Ale	500	170.0	0.0	14.0	1.70
Ghost Ship Pale Ale x 4	440	171.6	0.0	13.6	4.50
Spitfire Kentish Ale	500	185.0	0.0	13.5	1.25
Shepherd Neame Spitfire Premium Kentish Ale	500	185.0	0.0	15.5	1.25
Sainsbury's Suffolk Blonde Ale	500	190.0	0.0	15.5	1.80
Spitfire Gold Ale	500	190.0	0.0	15.5	1.83
Newcastle Brown Ale	550	220.0	0.0	17.1	1.38
Bishops Finger	500	225.0	0.0	17.5	1.25
Sainsbury's Kentish Ale, Taste the Difference	500	225.0	0.0	15.5	1.50
Wychwood Brewery Hobgoblin Ale	500	235.0	0.0	15.5	1.25
Hobgoblin	500	235.0	0.0	15.5	1.25
Wychwood Hobgoblin Extra Strong Ale	500	235.0	0.0	15.5	1.25
Black Sheep Ale	500	235.0	0.0	15.5	1.82
Sainsbury's India Pale Ale	500	255.0	0.0	15.5	1.50
Theakston Brewery Old Peculier Ale	500	260.0	0.0	25.5	1.83

Alcohol   Ale

Suggested Brands	Size (ml)	Kcal	S.fat (g)	Carbs (g)	£
Shepherd Neame 1698 Bottle Conditioned Ale	500	285.0	0.0	24.0	1.84

Values Shown Per Bottle Or Can (Price Per Individual Item)

Please Remember to Subscribe for the Latest Updates

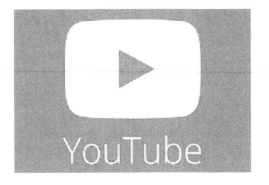

WWW.YOUTUBE.COM/STEPHENDBARNES

Bitter & Beers

Suggested Brands	Size (ml)	Kcal	S.fat (g)	Carbs (g)	£
M savers Bitter 2%	440	73	0	0	0.23
Bud Light Bottles	330	89	0	5	0.50
Corona	330	98	0	5	2.25
Morrisons Best Bitter	440	107	0	0	0.50
Budweiser alcohol free	330	111	0	26.5	0.75
Bud Light Cans	440	119	0	6.6	0.87
Boddingtons	440	132	0	0	0.93
John Smiths	440	132	0	0	0.94
Tetley's Original Bitter	440	145	0	11.9	0.77
Kronenbourg 1664	440	189	0	20.1	0.93
King Fisher	650	208	0	0	2.08
Cobra	620	248	0	18.7	1.93
Becks	620	257	0	18.6	1.76
Carlsberg Special Brew	440	304	0	0	1.88
Budweiser	660	317	0	21	1.95
Stella Artois Beer	660	320	0	13.1	1.76
Leffe	750	459	0	41	2.75

VALUES SHOWN PER BOTTLE OR CAN (PRICE PER INDIVIDUAL ITEM)

Cider

Suggested Brands	Size (ml)	Kcal	S.fat (g)	Carbs (g)	£
Waitrose Duchy Organic Herefordshire	500	125	0	0	1.67
Aspall Premier Cru Dry Suffolk Cider	500	137	0	18.0	1.76
Magners Original	440	162.7	0	8.8	0.67
Kopparberg Premium Cider with Mixed Fruits	400	168.5	0	30.3	2.03
Scrumpy Jack	440	185	0	17	1.00
Strongbow original	440	189	0	15.0	0.75
Thatchers Gold Somerset Cider	440	200	0	24	0.90
Average Cider Drink	440	210	0	23.3	1.00
Tesco Pear Cider	440	224	0	20.6	0.55
Bulmers Original Cider	500	238.6	0	25.8	0.94
Carling Cider	500	240	0	0	0.90
Stella Artois Cidre Apple Cider	500	352.1	1.4	56.3	1.00
Aspall medium cider	500	360.9	1.8	23.7	2.09
Strongbow Dark Fruit Cider	440	528	8.8	61.6	1.25

Values Shown Per Bottle Or Can (Price Per Individual Item)

Cocktails

Suggested Brands	Size (ml)	Kcal	S.fat (g)	Carbs (g)	£
Funkin Mojito	400	128.0	0.0	27.2	4.00
Funkin Bramble	400	288.0	0.0	71.6	4.00
Funkin Passion Fruit Martini	400	324.0	0.0	76.0	4.00
Daiquiri	250	475.0	0.0	17.8	1.00
Funkin Pina Colada	400	276.0	2.8	54.0	4.00

VALUES SHOWN PER DRINK

Your Favourite Food Not Included?
Let Us Know

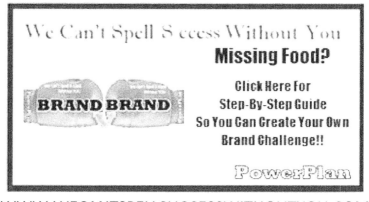

We Can't Spell Success Without You

Missing Food?

BRAND BRAND

Click Here For Step-By-Step Guide So You Can Create Your Own Brand Challenge!!

PowerPlan

WWW.WECANTSPELLSUCCESSWITHOUTYOU.COM

Larger

Suggested Brands	Size (ml)	Kcal	S.fat (g)	Carbs (g)	£
Becks	275	118	0	7.7	0.47
Red stripe	330	140	0	12.8	1.00
Carlsberg	440	141	0	8.8	0.84
Grolsch	330	142	0	6.9	0.83
Asahi	500	210	0	15	2.00
Fosters	440	227	0	17.6	0.90
Amstel	650	260	0	19.5	2.00
Staropramen	660	271	0	17.4	2.00
Peroni	500	273	0	29.8	2.70
San Miguel	660	288	0	0	1.49
San Niguel	660	288	0	0	2.00
Birra Moreetti	660	300	0	22	2.00
Tsingtao	330	314	0	28.6	2.00
Budweiser	660	317	0	21	1.95
Stella Artois Lager	660	320	0	13.1	1.76

VALUES SHOWN PER BOTTLE OR CAN (PRICE PER INDIVIDUAL ITEM)

Prosecco - Glass

Suggested Brands	Size	Kcal	S.fat (g)	Carbs (g)	£
Sainsbury's Prosecco Frizzante	75 cl	80	0	1.8	6.00
Sainsbury's Conegliano Prosecco, Taste the Difference	75 cl	82	0	1.8	8.00
Plaza Centro Prosecco	75 cl	84	0	1.8	5.00
Tesco Finest Prosecco Doc	75 cl	84	0	1.8	7.00
Morrisons The Best Valdobbiadene Prosecco 7	75 cl	84	0	1.8	10.00
Sainsbury's Prosecco DOC Extra Dry, SO Organi	75 cl	85	0	1.8	10.00
Bella Cucina Prosecco	75 cl	86	0	1.8	6.25
Prosecco Extra Dry	75 cl	93	0	1.8	6.00
Onbrina Prosecco Frizzante	75 cl	93	0	1.8	6.00
Canti Prosecco	75 cl	93	0	1.8	7.00
Fillipo Sansovino Prosecco	75 cl	93	0	1.8	7.00
Esatto Prosecco	75 cl	93	0	1.8	7.00
I Heart Prosecco	75 cl	93	0	1.8	7.00
Morrisons The Best Prosecco DOC	75 cl	93	0	1.8	7.00
Onbrina Prosecco	75 cl	93	0	1.8	7.00
Dandelione Prosecco	75 cl	93	0	1.8	7.95
ASDA Extra Special Prosecco Asolo Brut DOCG	75 cl	93	0	1.8	8.00
Pendium Prosecco	75 cl	93	0	1.8	8.50
Freixenet Prosecco D.O.C.	75 cl	93	0	1.8	9.00
Fillipo Sansovino Valdobbiadene Prosecco	75 cl	93	0	1.8	9.00

ALCOHOL   PROSECCO - GLASS

Suggested Brands	Size	Kcal	S.fat (g)	Carbs (g)	£
Alberto Nani Organic Prosecco	75 cl	93	0	1.8	9.00
Martini Prosecco	75 cl	93	0	1.8	10.00
Fillipo Sansovino Millesimato Brut Prosecco	75 cl	93	0	1.8	10.00
Echo Falls ProsEcho Falls Prosecco	75 cl	93	0	1.8	11.00
24KT Prosecco Brut	75 cl	93	0	1.8	12.00
Waitrose NV, Glera, Italian, Prosecco	75 cl	105	0	1.8	7.89
Sorso Prosecco Spumante 7	75 cl	143.8	0	1.8	6.00

VALUES SHOWN PER 125 ML GLASS

Prosecco - Bottle

Suggested Brands	Size	Kcal	S.fat (g)	Carbs (g)	£
Sainsbury's Prosecco Frizzante	75 cl	480	0.0	10.8	6.00
Sainsbury's Conegliano Prosecco, Taste the Difference	75 cl	492	0.0	10.8	8.00
Plaza Centro Prosecco	75 cl	504	0.0	10.8	5.00
Tesco Finest Prosecco Doc	75 cl	504	0.0	10.8	7.00
Morrisons The Best Valdobbiadene Prosecco 7	75 cl	504	0.0	10.8	10.00
Sainsbury's Prosecco DOC Extra Dry, SO Organi	75 cl	510	0.0	10.8	10.00
Bella Cucina Prosecco	75 cl	516	0.0	10.8	6.25
Prosecco Extra Dry	75 cl	558	0.0	10.8	6.00
Onbrina Prosecco Frizzante	75 cl	558	0.0	10.8	6.00
Canti Prosecco	75 cl	558	0.0	10.8	7.00
Fillipo Sansovino Prosecco	75 cl	558	0.0	10.8	7.00
Esatto Prosecco	75 cl	558	0.0	10.8	7.00
I Heart Prosecco	75 cl	558	0.0	10.8	7.00
Morrisons The Best Prosecco DOC	75 cl	558	0.0	10.8	7.00
Onbrina Prosecco	75 cl	558	0.0	10.8	7.00
Dandelione Prosecco	75 cl	558	0.0	10.8	7.95
ASDA Extra Special Prosecco Asolo Brut DOCG	75 cl	558	0.0	10.8	8.00
Pendium Prosecco	75 cl	558	0.0	10.8	8.50
Freixenet Prosecco D.O.C.	75 cl	558	0.0	10.8	9.00
Fillipo Sansovino Valdobbiadene Prosecco	75 cl	558	0.0	10.8	9.00

ALCOHOL   PROSECCO - BOTTLE

Suggested Brands	Size	Kcal	S.fat (g)	Carbs (g)	£
Alberto Nani Organic Prosecco	75 cl	558	0.0	10.8	9.00
Martini Prosecco	75 cl	558	0.0	10.8	10.00
Fillipo Sansovino Millesimato Brut Prosecco	75 cl	558	0.0	10.8	10.00
Echo Falls ProsEcho Falls Prosecco	75 cl	558	0.0	10.8	11.00
24KT Prosecco Brut	75 cl	558	0.0	10.8	12.00
Waitrose NV, Glera, Italian, Prosecco	75 cl	630	0.0	10.8	7.89
Sorso Prosecco Spumante	75 cl	863	0.0	10.8	6.00

VALUES SHOWN PER BOTTLE

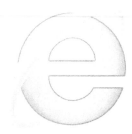

Find Us on The Web

WWW.WECANTSPELLSUCCESSWITHOUTYOU.COM

&

WWW.NADIET.INFO

Red Wine - Glass

Suggested Brands	Size	Kcal	S.fat (g)	Carbs (g)	£
Sainsbury's House Pinot Noir	75 cl	102.9	0.0	4.0	4.50
Tesco French Malbec	75 cl	110.3	0.0	3.5	5.00
Tesco Finest Cahors Malbec	75 cl	122.5	0.0	3.5	7.50
Tesco Finest Hawkes Bay Syrah	75 cl	122.5	0.0	4.4	10.00
Sainsbury's House Malbec	75 cl	124.3	0.0	3.5	4.50
Sainsbury's House Claret	75 cl	124.3	0.0	5.2	5.00
Tesco Finest Mercurey Pinot Noir	75 cl	124.3	0.0	0.9	14.00
Tesco Chilean Cabernet Sauvignon	75 cl	126	0.0	4.5	4.35
Sainsbury's House Cabernet Sauvignon	75 cl	126	0.0	4.5	4.40
Tesco Argentinian Malbec	75 cl	127.8	0.0	3.5	5.00
Sainsbury's Claret, Taste the Difference	75 cl	127.8	0.0	5.2	7.00
Tesco Claret	75 cl	129	0.0	5.2	5.00
Wm Morrison Malbec	75 cl	129.5	0.0	3.5	6.50
Sainsbury's Rheinhessen Pinot Noir, Taste the Difference	75 cl	129.5	0.0	4.0	6.75
Tesco Finest Argentinian Malbec	75 cl	129.5	0.0	3.5	8.00
Blossom Hill California red	75 cl	131.3	0.0	1.7	5.00
Morrisons Malbec	75 cl	131.3	0.0	3.5	5.00
Sainsbury's Cabernet Sauvignon, SO Organic	75 cl	131.3	0.0	4.5	6.50

ALCOHOL   RED WINE - GLASS

Suggested Brands	Size	Kcal	S.fat (g)	Carbs (g)	£
Tesco Finest Marlborough Pinot Noir	75 cl	131.3	0.0	0.9	8.00
Sainsbury's Chilean Pinot Noir, Taste the Difference	75 cl	131.3	0.0	4.0	8.50
Morrisons Pinot Noir	75 cl	131.5	0.0	4.0	4.75
Grignan-les-Adhémar Cuvée Traditionnelle	75 cl	132.4	0.0	4.1	5.00
Waitrose, Pinot Noir, Romanian	75 cl	133	0.0	4.0	5.99
Waitrose Argentinian Malbec	75 cl	133	0.0	3.5	7.99
Waitrose Maipo Valley Cabernet Sauvignon	75 cl	133	0.0	4.5	9.99
Sainsbury's Morador Malbec, Taste the Difference	75 cl	134.8	0.0	3.5	7.50
Morrisons The Best Malbec	75 cl	134.8	0.0	3.5	10.00
Tesco Finest The Trilogy Malbec	75 cl	134.8	0.0	3.5	10.50
Tesco Finest Angelica Sur Malbec	75 cl	134.8	0.0	3.5	18.00
Caminada Malbec	75 cl	136.5	0.0	3.5	5.00
Tesco Finest Maipo Cabernet Sauvignon	75 cl	136.5	0.0	4.5	10.50
Wm Morrison Cabernet Sauvignon	75 cl	138.3	0.0	4.5	6.00
Tesco Chilean Pinot Noir	75 cl	138.4	0.0	4.0	5.25
Morrisons Cabernet Sauvignon	75 cl	141.8	0.0	4.5	4.50

ALCOHOL RED WINE - GLASS

Suggested Brands	Size	Kcal	S.fat (g)	Carbs (g)	£
Sainsbury's Fairtrade Cabernet Sauvignon Merlot	75 cl	143.5	0.0	4.5	6.50
Winemaker's Choice Pinot Noir	75 cl	144.3	0.0	4.0	4.25
Bradshaw Pinot Noir	75 cl	144.3	0.0	4.0	5.50
Le Grand Clauzy Pinot Noir	75 cl	144.3	0.0	4.0	6.00
Morrison Chilean Pinot Noir	75 cl	144.3	0.0	4.0	7.00
Hans Baer Pinot Noir	75 cl	144.3	0.0	4.0	7.00
La Moneda Premium Collection Pinot Noir	75 cl	144.3	0.0	4.0	7.00
Cono Sur Pinot Noir	75 cl	144.3	0.0	4.0	7.50
Matua Pinot Noir	75 cl	144.3	0.0	4.0	8.00
Morrisons The Best Single Vineyard Pinot Noir	75 cl	144.3	0.0	4.0	9.00
ASDA Extra Special New Zealand Pinot Noir	75 cl	144.3	0.0	4.0	10.00
Errazuriz Wild Ferment Pinot Noir	75 cl	144.3	0.0	4.0	11.00
Villa Maria Pinot Noir Private Bin	75 cl	144.3	0.0	4.0	12.00
Wm Morrison Western Australia Cabernet Sauvignon	75 cl	145.3	0.0	4.5	6.50
The Wine List Merlot	75 cl	145.4	0.0	4.3	3.89
Vega Roja Merlot	75 cl	145.4	0.0	4.3	3.98
Hardys Classic Cabernet Merlot	75 cl	145.4	0.0	4.3	4.50

Suggested Brands	Size	Kcal	S.fat (g)	Carbs (g)	£
Southern Point Cabernet Sauvignon	75 cl	145.4	0.0	4.5	4.50
Flipflop Wines Merlot	75 cl	145.4	0.0	4.3	4.70
Etoile de Nuit Cabernet Sauvignon	75 cl	145.4	0.0	4.5	4.75
Winemaker's Choice Bordeaux Claret	75 cl	145.4	0.0	5.2	4.98
McGuigan Private Bin Merlot	75 cl	145.4	0.0	4.3	5.00
McGuigan Classic Merlot	75 cl	145.4	0.0	4.3	5.00
McGuigan Classic Cabernet Sauvignon	75 cl	145.4	0.0	4.5	5.00
Echo Falls Merlot	75 cl	145.4	0.0	4.3	5.25
Blossom Hill Merlot	75 cl	145.4	0.0	4.3	5.35
Barefoot Merlot	75 cl	145.4	0.0	4.3	5.50
Barefoot Cabernet Sauvignon	75 cl	145.4	0.0	4.5	5.50
Gallo Family Vineyards Merlot	75 cl	145.4	0.0	4.3	6.00
Casillero del Diablo Merlot	75 cl	145.4	0.0	4.3	6.00
Yellow Tail Merlot	75 cl	145.4	0.0	4.3	6.00
Lindeman's Cabernet Sauvignon Merlot	75 cl	145.4	0.0	4.3	6.00
ASDA Extra Special Cabernet Sauvignon	75 cl	145.4	0.0	4.5	6.00
McGuigan Reserve Cabernet Sauvignon	75 cl	145.4	0.0	4.5	6.00
McGuigan Black Label Merlot	75 cl	145.4	0.0	4.3	6.50
ASDA Extra Special Selection Syrah	75 cl	145.4	0.0	4.4	6.50

Suggested Brands	Size	Kcal	S.fat (g)	Carbs (g)	£
Errazuriz Merlot	75 cl	145.4	0.0	4.3	7.00
Hardys Nottage Hill Merlot	75 cl	145.4	0.0	4.3	7.00
Wolf Blass Yellow Label Cabernet Sauvignon	75 cl	145.4	0.0	4.5	7.00
Oyster Bay Hawkes Bay Merlot	75 cl	145.4	0.0	4.3	8.00
Les Chartrons, Bordeaux, French, Red Wine	75 cl	145.4	0.0	5.2	8.69
Château Les Martins Blaye Côtes de Bordeaux	75 cl	145.4	0.0	5.2	9.49
Burdizzo Chianti Riserva	75 cl	146.6	0.0	4.7	7.00
Echo Falls California Red	75 cl	147.8	0.0	4.5	5.99
ASDA Extra Special Barbera D'Asti	75 cl	149.0	0.0	4.8	6.50
Sainsbury's Malbec, SO Organic	75 cl	150.5	0.0	3.5	7.50
Quirky Bird Shiraz Mourvedre Viognier	75 cl	153.7	0.0	4.1	5.75
Zalze Shiraz Mourvedre Viognier	75 cl	153.7	0.0	4.1	7.50
Yalumba Y Series Shiraz Viognier	75 cl	153.7	0.0	4.1	8.50
Carnivor Zinfandel	75 cl	154.9	0.0	5.0	8.00
Red Fire Old Vine Zinfandel	75 cl	154.9	0.0	5.0	8.00
Winemaker's Choice Valle Central Malbec	75 cl	158	0.0	3.5	4.25
Gran Lomo Malbec	75 cl	158	0.0	3.5	5.00
Echo Falls Malbec	75 cl	158	0.0	3.5	5.00
Trivento Reserve Malbec	75 cl	158	0.0	3.5	6.00

ALCOHOL   RED WINE - GLASS

Suggested Brands	Size	Kcal	S.fat (g)	Carbs (g)	£
Tesco Finest Fair Trade South African Malbec	75 cl	158	0.0	3.5	6.00
Diversity of Terroir Premium Malbec	75 cl	158	0.0	3.5	6.50
Beefsteak Club Malbec, Argentinian	75 cl	158	0.0	3.5	6.74
Barefoot Malbec	75 cl	158	0.0	3.5	6.75
Rigal The Original Malbec	75 cl	158	0.0	3.5	7.00
La Moneda Premium Collection Malbec	75 cl	158	0.0	3.5	7.00
Wolf Blass Yellow Label Malbec	75 cl	158	0.0	3.5	7.00
ASDA Extra Special Malbec	75 cl	158	0.0	3.5	7.50
Luis Felipe Edwards Malbec	75 cl	158	0.0	3.5	7.50
Bodega Norton Barrel Select Malbec	75 cl	158	0.0	3.5	8.50
Bodega Norton Barrel Select Malbec	75 cl	158	0.0	3.5	8.50
Dark Horse Malbec	75 cl	158	0.0	3.5	8.50
Trapiche Finca Las Palmas Malbec	75 cl	158	0.0	3.5	12.00
Trivento Golden Reserve Malbec	75 cl	158	0.0	3.5	16.00
Tesco Finest Central Otago Pinot Noir	75 cl	180.3	0.0	4.0	13.00

VALUES SHOWN PER 175 ML GLASS

Red Wine - Bottle

Suggested Brands	Size	Kcal	S.fat (g)	Carbs (g)	£
Sainsbury's House Pinot Noir	75 cl	441.0	0.0	17.1	4.50
Tesco French Malbec	75 cl	472.7	0.0	15.0	5.00
Tesco Finest Cahors Malbec	75 cl	525.0	0.0	15.0	7.50
Tesco Finest Hawkes Bay Syrah	75 cl	525.0	0.0	18.9	10.00
Sainsbury's House Malbec	75 cl	532.7	0.0	15.0	4.50
Sainsbury's House Claret	75 cl	532.7	0.0	22.3	5.00
Tesco Finest Mercurey Pinot Noir	75 cl	532.7	0.0	3.9	14.00
Tesco Chilean Cabernet Sauvignon	75 cl	540.0	0.0	19.3	4.35
Sainsbury's House Cabernet Sauvignon	75 cl	540.0	0.0	19.3	4.40
Tesco Argentinian Malbec	75 cl	547.7	0.0	15.0	5.00
Sainsbury's Claret, Taste the Difference	75 cl	547.7	0.0	22.3	7.00
Tesco Claret	75 cl	552.9	0.0	22.3	5.00
Wm Morrison Malbec	75 cl	555.0	0.0	15.0	6.50
Sainsbury's Rheinhessen Pinot Noir, Taste the Difference	75 cl	555.0	0.0	17.1	6.75
Tesco Finest Argentinian Malbec	75 cl	555.0	0.0	15.0	8.00
Blossom Hill California red	75 cl	562.7	0.0	7.3	5.00
Morrisons Malbec	75 cl	562.7	0.0	15.0	5.00
Sainsbury's Cabernet Sauvignon, SO Organic	75 cl	562.7	0.0	19.3	6.50

Suggested Brands	Size	Kcal	S.fat (g)	Carbs (g)	£
Tesco Finest Marlborough Pinot Noir	75 cl	562.7	0.0	3.9	8.00
Sainsbury's Chilean Pinot Noir, Taste the Difference	75 cl	562.7	0.0	17.1	8.50
Morrisons Pinot Noir	75 cl	563.6	0.0	17.1	4.75
Grignan-les-Adhémar Cuvée Traditionnelle	75 cl	567.4	0.0	17.6	5.00
Waitrose, Pinot Noir, Romanian	75 cl	570.0	0.0	17.1	5.99
Waitrose Argentinian Malbec	75 cl	570.0	0.0	15.0	7.99
Waitrose Maipo Valley Cabernet Sauvignon	75 cl	570.0	0.0	19.3	9.99
Sainsbury's Morador Malbec, Taste the Difference	75 cl	577.7	0.0	15.0	7.50
Morrisons The Best Malbec	75 cl	577.7	0.0	15.0	10.00
Tesco Finest The Trilogy Malbec	75 cl	577.7	0.0	15.0	10.50
Tesco Finest Angelica Sur Malbec	75 cl	577.7	0.0	15.0	18.00
Caminada Malbec	75 cl	585.0	0.0	15.0	5.00
Tesco Finest Maipo Cabernet Sauvignon	75 cl	585.0	0.0	19.3	10.50
Wm Morrison Cabernet Sauvignon	75 cl	592.7	0.0	19.3	6.00
Tesco Chilean Pinot Noir	75 cl	593.1	0.0	17.1	5.25
Morrisons Cabernet Sauvignon	75 cl	607.7	0.0	19.3	4.50

ALCOHOL RED WINE - BOTTLE

Suggested Brands	Size	Kcal	S.fat (g)	Carbs (g)	£
Sainsbury's Fairtrade Cabernet Sauvignon Merlot	75 cl	615.0	0.0	19.3	6.50
Winemaker's Choice Pinot Noir	75 cl	618.4	0.0	17.1	4.25
Bradshaw Pinot Noir	75 cl	618.4	0.0	17.1	5.50
Le Grand Clauzy Pinot Noir	75 cl	618.4	0.0	17.1	6.00
Morrison Chilean Pinot Noir	75 cl	618.4	0.0	17.1	7.00
Hans Baer Pinot Noir	75 cl	618.4	0.0	17.1	7.00
La Moneda Premium Collection Pinot Noir	75 cl	618.4	0.0	17.1	7.00
Cono Sur Pinot Noir	75 cl	618.4	0.0	17.1	7.50
Matua Pinot Noir	75 cl	618.4	0.0	17.1	8.00
Morrisons The Best Single Vineyard Pinot Noir	75 cl	618.4	0.0	17.1	9.00
ASDA Extra Special New Zealand Pinot Noir	75 cl	618.4	0.0	17.1	10.00
Errazuriz Wild Ferment Pinot Noir	75 cl	618.4	0.0	17.1	11.00
Villa Maria Pinot Noir Private Bin	75 cl	618.4	0.0	17.1	12.00
Wm Morrison Western Australia Cabernet Sauvignon	75 cl	622.7	0.0	19.3	6.50
The Wine List Merlot	75 cl	623.1	0.0	18.4	3.89
Vega Roja Merlot	75 cl	623.1	0.0	18.4	3.98
Hardys Classic Cabernet Merlot	75 cl	623.1	0.0	18.4	4.50

ALCOHOL RED WINE - BOTTLE

Suggested Brands	Size	Kcal	S.fat (g)	Carbs (g)	£
Southern Point Cabernet Sauvignon	75 cl	623.1	0.0	19.3	4.50
Flipflop Wines Merlot	75 cl	623.1	0.0	18.4	4.70
Etoile de Nuit Cabernet Sauvignon	75 cl	623.1	0.0	19.3	4.75
Winemaker's Choice Bordeaux Claret	75 cl	623.1	0.0	22.3	4.98
McGuigan Private Bin Merlot	75 cl	623.1	0.0	18.4	5.00
McGuigan Classic Merlot	75 cl	623.1	0.0	18.4	5.00
McGuigan Classic Cabernet Sauvignon	75 cl	623.1	0.0	19.3	5.00
Echo Falls Merlot	75 cl	623.1	0.0	18.4	5.25
Blossom Hill Merlot	75 cl	623.1	0.0	18.4	5.35
Barefoot Merlot	75 cl	623.1	0.0	18.4	5.50
Barefoot Cabernet Sauvignon	75 cl	623.1	0.0	19.3	5.50
Gallo Family Vineyards Merlot	75 cl	623.1	0.0	18.4	6.00
Casillero del Diablo Merlot	75 cl	623.1	0.0	18.4	6.00
Yellow Tail Merlot	75 cl	623.1	0.0	18.4	6.00
Lindeman's Cabernet Sauvignon Merlot	75 cl	623.1	0.0	18.4	6.00
ASDA Extra Special Cabernet Sauvignon	75 cl	623.1	0.0	19.3	6.00
McGuigan Reserve Cabernet Sauvignon	75 cl	623.1	0.0	19.3	6.00
McGuigan Black Label Merlot	75 cl	623.1	0.0	18.4	6.50

Suggested Brands	Size	Kcal	S.fat (g)	Carbs (g)	£
ASDA Extra Special Selection Syrah	75 cl	623.1	0.0	18.9	6.50
Errazuriz Merlot	75 cl	623.1	0.0	18.4	7.00
Hardys Nottage Hill Merlot	75 cl	623.1	0.0	18.4	7.00
Wolf Blass Yellow Label Cabernet Sauvignon	75 cl	623.1	0.0	19.3	7.00
Oyster Bay Hawkes Bay Merlot	75 cl	623.1	0.0	18.4	8.00
Les Chartrons, Bordeaux, French, Red Wine	75 cl	623.1	0.0	22.3	8.69
Château Les Martins Blaye Côtes de Bordeaux	75 cl	623.1	0.0	22.3	9.49
Burdizzo Chianti Riserva	75 cl	628.3	0.0	20.1	7.00
Echo Falls California Red	75 cl	633.4	0.0	19.3	5.99
ASDA Extra Special Barbera D'Asti	75 cl	638.6	0.0	20.6	6.50
Sainsbury's Malbec, SO Organic	75 cl	645.0	0.0	15.0	7.50
Quirky Bird Shiraz Mourvedre Viognier	75 cl	658.7	0.0	17.6	5.75
Zalze Shiraz Mourvedre Viognier	75 cl	658.7	0.0	17.6	7.50
Yalumba Y Series Shiraz Viognier	75 cl	658.7	0.0	17.6	8.50
Carnivor Zinfandel	75 cl	663.9	0.0	21.4	8.00
Red Fire Old Vine Zinfandel	75 cl	663.9	0.0	21.4	8.00
Winemaker's Choice Valle Central Malbec	75 cl	677.1	0.0	15.0	4.25
Gran Lomo Malbec	75 cl	677.1	0.0	15.0	5.00

ALCOHOL   RED WINE - BOTTLE

Suggested Brands	Size	Kcal	S.fat (g)	Carbs (g)	£
Echo Falls Malbec	75 cl	677.1	0.0	15.0	5.00
Trivento Reserve Malbec	75 cl	677.1	0.0	15.0	6.00
Tesco Finest Fair Trade South African Malbec	75 cl	677.1	0.0	15.0	6.00
Diversity of Terroir Premium Malbec	75 cl	677.1	0.0	15.0	6.50
Beefsteak Club Malbec, Argentinian	75 cl	677.1	0.0	15.0	6.74
Barefoot Malbec	75 cl	677.1	0.0	15.0	6.75
Rigal The Original Malbec	75 cl	677.1	0.0	15.0	7.00
La Moneda Premium Collection Malbec	75 cl	677.1	0.0	15.0	7.00
Wolf Blass Yellow Label Malbec	75 cl	677.1	0.0	15.0	7.00
ASDA Extra Special Malbec	75 cl	677.1	0.0	15.0	7.50
Luis Felipe Edwards Malbec	75 cl	677.1	0.0	15.0	7.50
Bodega Norton Barrel Select Malbec	75 cl	677.1	0.0	15.0	8.50
Bodega Norton Barrel Select Malbec	75 cl	677.1	0.0	15.0	8.50
Dark Horse Malbec	75 cl	677.1	0.0	15.0	8.50
Trapiche Finca Las Palmas Malbec	75 cl	677.1	0.0	15.0	12.00
Trivento Golden Reserve Malbec	75 cl	677.1	0.0	15.0	16.00
Tesco Finest Central Otago Pinot Noir	75 cl	772.7	0.0	17.1	13.00

VALUES SHOWN PER BOTTLE

Spirits - Bourbon

Suggested Brands	Size (cl)	Kcal	S.fat (g)	Carbs (g)	£
Pims	70cl	64	0	1.6	15.30
Jim Beam White Label Bourbon	70 cl	87	0	0	14.00
ASDA Blended Bourbon	70 cl	87	0	0	14.00
Old Samuel Blended Bourbon Whisky	70 cl	87	0	0	14.35
Jack Daniels Tennessee Fire	70 cl	87	0	0	16.00
Buffalo Trace Bourbon Whiskey	70 cl	87	0	0	23.00
Maker's Mark Kentucky Straight Bourbon Whisky	70 cl	87	0	0	25.00
Bulleit Bourbon Frontier Whiskey	70 cl	87	0	0	27.00
Sainsbury's Honey Bourbon Liqueur	70 cl	100	0	0	13.50
Sainsbury's Kentucky Bourbon Whiskey	70 cl	101	0	0	13.50

VALUES SHOWN PER 40 ML SHOT

Spirits - Brandy

Suggested Brands	Size (cl)	Kcal	S.fat (g)	Carbs (g)	£
Tesco Napoleon Brandy	1 L	80	0	0	16.00
Tesco Finest Xo Brandy	70 cl	80	0	0	16.50
Waitrose 3 Year Old French Brandy	70 cl	81	0	0	13.25
Waitrose 3 Year Old French Brandy	1 L	81	0	0	17.50
Tesco Spanish Brandy	70 cl	82	0	0	14.50
ASDA Napoleon French V.S.O.P. Brandy	70cl	87	0	0	11.50
Morrisons 3 Year Old French Brandy	70 cl	87	0	0	12.50
Jules Clairon Fine French Brandy	70cl	87	0	0	13.50
Soberano 5 Brandy Reserva	70 cl	87	0	0	14.00
ASDA Napoleon French V.S.O.P. Brandy	1 L	87	0	0	16.00
ASDA Extra Special Rare Old French XO Brandy	70 cl	87	0	0	16.00
Sainsbury's 3 Year Old French Brandy	1 L	87	0	0	16.00
M Best Brandy XO	70 cl	87	0	0	16.00
EJ Brandy Original Brandy	70 cl	87	0	0	16.50
Three Barrels Rare Old French Brandy VSOP	1 L	87	0	0	19.00
Bardinet Brandy	1 L	87	0	0	19.00

VALUES SHOWN PER 40 ML SHOT

Spirits - Gin

Suggested Brands	Size (cl)	Kcal	S.fat (g)	Carbs (g)	£
Gin Gordons	1 L	52	0	0	16.00
Sainsbury's Dry Gin	1 L	82	0	0	15.40
Sainsbury's Gin,	70 cl	83	0	0	10.00
Waitrose London Dry Gin	1 L	83	0	0	16.35
Tesco Dry London Gin	1 L	86	0	0	15.00
Gin Bombay Sapphire	1 L	94.4	0	0	20.00
Sainsbury's Blackfriars Gin, Taste the Difference	70 cl	95	0	0	16.00
M Best Gin	70 cl	99	0	0	16.00
Ungava Canadian Premium Gin	29.5	99	0	0	27.00
Morrisons London Dry Gin	70 cl	107	0	0	11.00
ASDA London Dry Gin	1 L	107	0	0	14.95
Bombay London Dry Gin	1 L	107	0	0	16.00
Tanqueray London Dry Gin	70 cl	107	0	0	16.00
Opihr Oriental Spiced London Dry Gin	70 cl	107	0	0	18.00
Gordon's Sloe Gin	70 cl	133	0	0	15.00

VALUES SHOWN PER 40 ML SHOT

Spirits - Rum

Suggested Brands	Size (cl)	Kcal	S.fat (g)	Carbs (g)	£
Malibu Original White Rum	1 L	81.6	0	0	20.00
Sainsbury's Superior Dark Rum	1 L	83	0	0	15.40
Sainsbury's Superior White Rum	1 L	83	0	0	15.40
Bacardi white rum	70cl	86	0	10	16.50
Tesco Coconut Rum	70 cl	87	0	0	8.00
ASDA Fine Dark Navy Rum	70 cl	87	0	0	11.00
Tesco Spiced Gold Rum	70 cl	87	0	0	11.87
Lamb's Navy Rum	70 cl	87	0	0	14.00
Havana Club 3 Year Old White Rum	70 cl	87	0	0	15.00
Bacardí Spiced Premium Spirit Rum	70 cl	87	0	0	15.00
ASDA Refined Dark Navy Rum	1 L	87	0	0	15.00
ASDA Carta Blanc Superior White Rum	1 L	87	0	0	15.00
Tesco Dark Rum	1 L	87	0	0	15.00
Tesco White Rum	1 L	87	0	0	15.00
Bacardi Carta Blanca Rum	70 cl	87	0	0	16.00
Sailor Jerry Spiced Rum	70cl	87	0	0	16.00
Captain Morgan Rum	70 cl	87	0	0	16.25
Mount Gay 1703 Eclipse Rum	70cl	87	0	0	17.50
The Kraken Black Spiced Rum	70 cl	87	0	0	20.00
Red Leg Spiced Rum	70 cl	87	0	0	20.00

Alcohol Spirits - Rum

Suggested Brands	Size (cl)	Kcal	S.fat (g)	Carbs (g)	£
Havana Club Añejo Especial Rum	70 cl	87	0	0	20.50
Wood's 100 Navy Rum	70 cl	87	0	0	22.50
Havana Club 7 Year Old Dark Rum	70 cl	87	0	0	26.00
Wray & Nephew White Overproof Rum	70 cl	87	0	0	26.00
The Duppy Share Caribbean Rum	70 cl	87	0	0	26.00
Kirk & Sweeney 12 Year Old Rum	70 cl	87	0	0	32.00

Values Shown Per 40 ml Shot

Find Us On

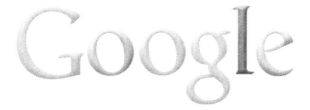

Search: **NADIET.INFO**

Spirits - Vodka

Suggested Brands	Size	Kcal	S.fat (g)	Carbs (g)	£
Smirnoff Red Label Vodka	70cl	73	0	0	15.00
Sainsbury's Vodka, Basics	70cl	82.4	0	0	10.00
Sainsbury's Vodka	1L	82.4	0	0	15.40
Morrisons Imperial Vodka	70cl	82.8	0	0	11.00
Waitrose Vodka	70cl	83.2	0	0	12.49
Glen's Vodka	70cl	87	0	0	13.50
ASDA Triple Distilled Vodka	1L	87	0	0	14.95
Russian Standard Vodka	70cl	87	0	0	15.00
Vladivar Vodka	1L	87	0	0	15.50
Russian Standard Vodka	1L	87	0	0	16.00
Wm Morrison Vodka	70cl	87	0	0	16.00
Absolut Original Swedish Vodka	29.5 ml	87	0	0	19.00
Russian Standard Gold Vodka	70cl	87	0	0	23.50

VALUES SHOWN PER 40 ML SHOT

Spirits - Whiskey

Suggested Brands	Size	Kcal	S.fat (g)	Carbs (g)	£
Sainsbury's Scotch Whisky, Basics	70cl	88	0	0	11.00
Tesco Special Reserve Scotch Whisky	1L	89	0	0	16.30
Waitrose Blended Scotch Whisky	1L	89	0	0	18.49
Jack Daniel's Old No. 7 Tennessee Whiskey	70cl	90	0	0	16.00
Morrisons Scotch Whisky	70cl	95	0	0	12.00
High Commissioner Blended Scotch Whisky	70cl	95	0	0	13.50
The Famous Grouse Blended Scotch Whisky	1L	95	0	0	16.00
Whyte & Mackay Blended Scotch Whisky	1L	95	0	0	16.00
Sainsbury's Blended Whisky	1L	95	0	0	16.00
Sainsbury's Speyside Whisky, Taste the Difference	70cl	95	0	0	18.00
Johnnie Walker Red Label Blended Scotch Whisky	70cl	95	0	0	18.00
ASDA Extra Special Islay Single Malt Scotch Whisky	70cl	95	0	0	18.50
Glenfairn Islay Single Malt Whisky	70cl	95	0	0	20.00
Glen Moray Speyside Single Malt Scotch Whisky	70cl	95	0	0	20.00
Bells Original Original	1L	95	0	0	20.50

Suggested Brands	Size	Kcal	S.fat (g)	Carbs (g)	£
ASDA McKendrick's Blended Scotch Whisky 3 Years Old	1.5L	95	0	0	23.62
Jameson Irish Whiskey	1L	95	0	0	25.00
Cardhu Gold Reserve Single Malt Whisky	70cl	95	0	0	26.00
Bulleit Bourbon Frontier Whiskey	70cl	95	0	0	27.00

Values Shown Per 40 ml Shot

Stout

Suggested Brands	Size (g)	Kcal	S.fat (g)	Carbs (g)	£
Guinness Foreign Extra Stout	330	215	0	16.5	1.83
Big Drop Low Alcohol Stout	330	91	0.3	17.8	1.30
Black Sheep Choc & Orange Stout	500	280	0.5	27	1.80
Guinness Original Stout	500	185	9	4.4	1.70

Values Shown Per Bottle Or Can (Price Per Individual Item)

White Wine - Glass

Suggested Brands	Size (g)	Kcal	S.fat (g)	Carbs (g)	£
Lindeman's Alcohol Free Chardonnay Pinot Nior Muscat	75 cl	22.8	0.0	4.7	3.98
Lindeman's Alcohol Free Semillon Chardonnay	75 cl	26.3	0.0	5.3	3.98
Black Tower	75 cl	77.0	0.0	6.9	5.00
ASDA Extra Special Muscat	75 cl	87.5	0.0	17.5	2.50
Sainsbury's House Pinot Grigio	75 cl	117.1	0.0	5.4	4.50
Echo Falls Medium White	75 cl	141.9	0.0	17.7	4.00
Kumala Chenin Blanc	75 cl	141.9	0.0	5.8	4.25
Dr. Loosen Bros Riesling Dry	75 cl	141.9	0.0	6.5	7.00
Bradshaw Sauvignon Blanc	75 cl	143.1	0.0	3.5	4.75
Touraine Sauvignon Blanc	75 cl	143.1	0.0	3.5	8.00
Calvet Alsace Pinot Blanc	75 cl	143.1	0.0	3.3	9.00
Villa Maria Sauvignon Blanc Marlborough	75 cl	143.1	0.0	3.5	9.50
Lindeman's Tollana Chardonnay	75 cl	144.3	0.0	4.0	4.50
Hardys Stamp of Australia Chardonnay Semillon	75 cl	144.3	0.0	5.3	5.50
Hardys Stamp of Australia Sauvignon Semillon	75 cl	144.3	0.0	5.3	5.50
Busby Estate Margaret River Sauvignon Blanc Semillon	75 cl	144.3	0.0	5.3	5.50

Suggested Brands	Size (g)	Kcal	S.fat (g)	Carbs (g)	£
Wolf Blass Red Label Chardonnay Semillon	75 cl	144.3	0.0	5.3	6.00
Table Wine	75 cl	144.3	0.0	4.5	7.50
ASDA Extra Special Pouilly Fume Sauvignon Blanc	75 cl	144.3	0.0	3.9	12.50
Blossom Hill	75 cl	157.3	0.0	1.8	5.00

Values Shown Per 175 ml Glass

Your Favourite Food Not Included?
Let Us Know

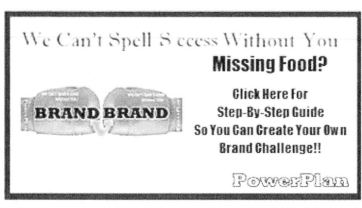

WWW.WECANTSPELLSUCCESSWITHOUTYOU.COM

White Wine - Bottle

Suggested Brands	Size (g)	Kcal	S.fat (g)	Carbs (g)	£
Lindeman's Alcohol Free Chardonnay Pinot Nior Muscat	75 cl	97.5	0.0	20.1	3.98
Lindeman's Alcohol Free Semillon Chardonnay	75 cl	112.5	0.0	22.5	3.98
Black Tower	75 cl	330.0	0.0	29.6	5.00
ASDA Extra Special Muscat	75 cl	375	0.0	75.0	2.50
Sainsbury's House Pinot Grigio	75 cl	501.9	0.0	23.1	4.50
Echo Falls Medium White	75 cl	608.1	0.0	75.9	4.00
Kumala Chenin Blanc	75 cl	608.1	0.0	24.9	4.25
Dr. Loosen Bros Riesling Dry	75 cl	608.1	0.0	27.9	7.00
Bradshaw Sauvignon Blanc	75 cl	613.3	0.0	15.0	4.75
Touraine Sauvignon Blanc	75 cl	613.3	0.0	15.0	8.00
Calvet Alsace Pinot Blanc	75 cl	613.3	0.0	14.1	9.00
Villa Maria Sauvignon Blanc Marlborough	75 cl	613.3	0.0	15.0	9.50
Lindeman's Tollana Chardonnay	75 cl	618.4	0.0	17.1	4.50
Hardys Stamp of Australia Chardonnay Semillon	75 cl	618.4	0.0	22.7	5.50
Hardys Stamp of Australia Sauvignon Semillon	75 cl	618.4	0.0	22.7	5.50
Busby Estate Margaret River Sauvignon Blanc Semillon	75 cl	618.4	0.0	22.7	5.50

ALCOHOL　WHITE WINE - BOTTLE

Suggested Brands	Size (g)	Kcal	S.fat (g)	Carbs (g)	£
Wolf Blass Red Label Chardonnay Semillon	75 cl	618.4	0.0	22.7	6.00
Table Wine	75 cl	618.4	0.0	19.3	7.50
ASDA Extra Special Pouilly Fume Sauvignon Blanc	75 cl	618.4	0.0	16.7	12.50
Blossom Hill	75 cl	674.1	0.0	7.7	5.00

VALUES SHOWN PER BOTTLE

Final Word from the Author

If you are having a health or weight issue for the first time, then changing your lifestyle using habits is a great idea rather than using one of the many diets available. These fad diets simply make your weight yo-yo, this only improves your health over a short time as a diet is difficult, and generally too expensive, to maintain for life.

Using the brand versus brand range of books and habits will allow you to control your weight, lower your chances of suffering from heart and cholesterol issues and will allow you to escape the diabetes type 2 condition. Alternatively, using the super money saver edition will also help you to increase your bank balance and enjoy life to the max!

Do not forget to visit our website WWW.NADIET.INFO where you can email your feedback regarding this brand versus brand book and see the latest food fact sheets for 2020 and beyond.

I always appreciate your support, once again thank you for purchasing this book and sharing in our ideas.

Wishing you all the success and happiness in the world as you celebrate the new you!

Regards,

Stephen D. Barnes

Glossary

Term	Definition	Page
HDL	**High-Density Lipoprotein Cholesterol** The amount of good fats stored in the body shown in the results of a blood test. The higher the level of H.D.L the healthier the body becomes. If low levels are indicated than this is considered a major risk factor for heart disease.	161
LDL	**Low-Density Lipoprotein Cholesterol** The amount of bad fats stored in the body shown in the results of a blood test. The higher the level of L.D.L the more likely you will have increased fat in the arteries leading to poor health.	161
IBS	**Irritable Bowel Syndrome** A common disorder that affects the large intestine.	351

References

Asda Website
Free to use website showing food that the store sells in the UK. This also tends to show calorie and nutrition information that has been used in this book.
www.asda.com

Tesco Website
Free to use website showing food that the store sells in the UK. This also tends to show calorie and nutrition information that has been used in this book.
www.tesco.com

Morrison's Website
Free to use website showing food that the store sells in the UK. This also tends to show calorie and nutrition information that has been used in this book.

I did notice that many of the M saver products are not listed on the supermarket's website, if this book quotes an M saver product then the information has been taken directly from the packaging.
www.sainsburys.co.uk

Sainsbury's Website
Free to use website showing food that the store sells in the UK. This also tends to show calorie and nutrition information that has been used in this book.

I did notice that many of the Sainsbury's products are misspelt, the actual website spelling is duplicated in this book without correction.
www.groceries.morrisons.com

Waitrose Website

Free to use website showing food that the store sells in the UK. This also tends to show calorie and nutrition information that has been used in this book.

www.waitrose.com

Iceland Website

Free to use website showing food that the store sells in the UK. This also tends to show calorie and nutrition information that has been used in this book.

www.iceland.co.uk

Aldi & Lidl

Most of the products at these stores are available on the supermarkets website BUT without calorie and nutrition information. If this book quotes an Aldi or Lidl product then the information has been taken directly from the packaging.

www.aldi.co.uk

www.lidl.co.uk

Samsung Health

A free phone app and a method of monitoring the body intake of calories by logging food and daily activities performed by the body. The body can be monitored when wearing the Samsung Gear S3 watch, this is extremely accurate when checking heartbeat and the number of steps walked.

The app also provides calorie and nutrition information that proved very useful when creating this book.

www.samsung.com/uk/samsung-health

My Fitness Pal

A free phone app used to monitor the amount of food consumed daily by scanning the barcode on the packaging. A supported website discloses food nutrition that is also useful for calorie counting.

www.myfitnesspal.com

Google

Internet search engine that is very useful for researching projects. This website proved very useful when researching calorie and nutrition information when not shown on supermarket websites or food packaging.

www.google.co.uk

Credits

Picture of Fish
Free image download and used in this publication from
www.needpix.com
Pg 166

Picture of Chicken Nuggets
Free image download and used in this publication from
www.commons.wikimedia.org.com
Pg 224

Picture of Good Morning Coffee
Free image download and used in this publication from
www.needpix.com
Pg 356

Also Available

We Can't Spell S ccess

Finally Control
Weight For Life

**Convenient Regular
Exercise Instantly**

How To Escape
From Diabetes

Without

YOU

Goodbye
To Diets

Hello To

Habits

*Gold
Edition*

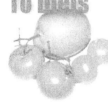

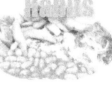

PowerPlan

Witten By Stephen D. Barnes

My Ultimate Self Help Book

We Can't Spell S ccess

Finally Control Weight For Life   **Convenient Regular Exercise Instantly**   **How To Escape From Diabetes**

Without

YOU

Goodbye To Diets   **Hello To Habits**

Silver Edition

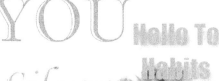

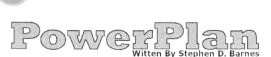

Witten By Stephen D. Barnes

My Ultimate Self Help Book

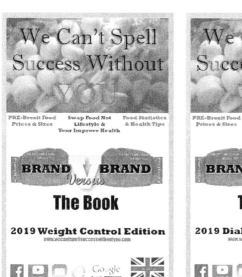

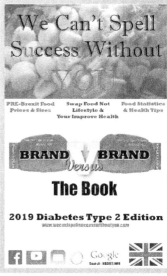

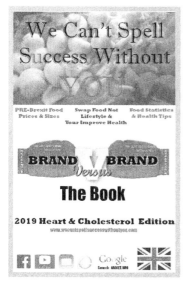

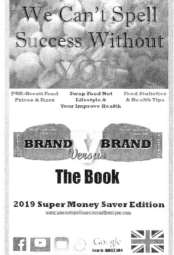

Printed in Great Britain
by Amazon